Family
Aromatherapy

JOAN RADFORD

foulsham

LONDON • NEW YORK • TORONTO • SYDNEY

foulsham

The Publishing House, Bennetts Close, Cippenham,
Slough, Berkshire, SL1 5AP, England

To Peter, with all my love. Also in loving memory of my dear friends,
Caroline Lindop and Laurence Baine. My thanks to Bernie Hephrun,
Pat Drummond, Ann Mathias, Pat Fuller and Eileen Lloyd for their help.

ISBN 0-572-02436-3
Copyright © 1999 Joan Radford

Neither the editors of W. Foulsham & Co. Limited nor the
author or the publisher take responsibility for any possible
consequences from any treatment, procedure, test exercise,
action, or application of medicine or preparation by any person
reading or following the information in this book. The
publication does not constitute the practice of medicine, and
this book does not attempt to replace your doctor. The authors
and publisher advise the reader to check with a doctor before
administering any medication or undertaking any course of
treatment or exercise.

Typeset in Great Britain by Grafica, Bournemouth
Printed in Great Britain by St. Edmundsbury Press Ltd,
Bury St. Edmunds, Suffolk

Contents

Introduction

*A*ROMATHERAPY is the use of essential oils for their
therapeutic properties. An essential oil is a highly
odiferous substance found in particular aromatic plants. The oil
usually bears the name of the plant from which it is derived, for
example jasmine or lavender, though there are a number of
exceptions, such as neroli, which is extracted from orange
blossom. The oil is stored as microdroplets in tiny sacs or
glands. According to the species, essential oil is obtained from
the flowers, leaves, stems, roots, fruits or seeds, and sometimes
from the whole plant. Certain barks and woods are a source,
yielding gums and resins from which the essential oil is
extracted by distillation.

Essential oils are not greasy like vegetable oils (for example
olive, corn, soya). They are light, volatile and made
up of complex mixtures of organic chemicals (acids, esters,
alcohols, aldehydes, ketones, terpenes and phenols).

Every essential oil used in aromatherapy has its own specific
healing properties. Most of the oils are antiseptic to some
degree, and will combat micro-organisms. A number of the
oils can be used to calm the nervous system, others reduce
inflammation, or ease aches and pains, benefit particular
organs and systems of the body, uplift the spirits – the list could
go on and on.

Essential oils are usually diluted and applied to the skin, or inhaled. However, some schools of aromatherapy advocate taking essential oils internally. There is considerable controversy surrounding this. Personally, I think it is safer not to ingest essential oils unless directed by a qualified herbalist or medical practitioner. External application and inhalation are usually considered faster and more effective methods of use than ingestion. Mouthwashes or gargles are also safe, provided they are not swallowed.

An important characteristic of essential oils is that they quickly penetrate the layers of the skin and enter the bloodstream. They are therefore fast-acting. But the oils are very strong and not generally applied undiluted to the skin. As they readily dissolve in fatty vegetable oils (not in water), they are conveniently used in massage oils, creams and lotions. Clinical tests have shown that essential oils enter the bloodstream more quickly by inhalation than either through the skin or orally.

Aromatherapy at Home

Using aromatherapy at home for yourself, your family and friends has considerable advantages. For a start, it will be cheaper than going for professional treatment, although the benefits of this should not be dismissed – there are times when it is essential to consult a professional aromatherapist. Being able to carry out treatments at home is much more convenient than having to wait, sometimes several weeks, for an appointment with an aromatherapist. When you feel a symptom coming on, treatment can be immediate. The axiom 'prevention is better than cure' is a very good reason for such self-help. Always consult your GP for persistent symptoms and in cases of pain, swelling or fever.

You can do away with most of those proprietary medicines from the chemist – for coughs and colds, sinusitis, sore throats, headaches and so on. Nor will you need to buy special skin creams, anti-cellulite lotions, air-fresheners, disinfectants and antiseptics: aromatherapy can provide all of these.

The use of essential oils has a marked effect on the health of the skin. It would be blatantly dishonest for me to claim that aromatherapy can work miracles, reversing the ravages of time. However, I will state positively that essential oils can improve the tone and general condition of the skin and, if used regularly from about the age of 20, the effects of the ageing process can be delayed.

Unlike modern drugs and medicines, the essential oils generally used in aromatherapy rarely have unpleasant side effects. Instead, they help bring about harmony and well-being, peace and tranquillity. This book tells you how to use essential oils effectively and safely.

In cases of anxiety, depression, tension and stress, essential oils are much safer than chemical tranquillisers or stimulants. The oils tend to be normalising or balancing rather than directly stimulating or sedating. Being of an organic, subtle nature, they act in similarly subtle and complex ways.

It takes a skilled professional aromatherapist to be able to select the best blend of oils for an individual. Not only will the therapist have a thorough knowledge of the effects of different oils on specific parts of the body, the psychological state of the client will be a major consideration too. A good training course and experience gathered over years of practice are necessary for anyone wishing to acquire a high degree of expertise, but anyone, with the aid of this book, can learn enough of the basics of aromatherapy to be able to tackle most minor disorders, injuries and psychological conditions. Knowing that one has an instant and effective remedy at hand is very comforting. I occasionally come across differing reactions to certain oils, but the well-tried formulas you'll find in this book work well for most people.

Always be sensible with your health. If symptoms persist or you are not certain about their cause, consult a doctor.

Orthodox medication does not interfere with the efficacy of aromatherapy treatments, or vice versa. Indeed, medical treatment and aromatherapy can help one another (but note cautions on pages 49–56). Homoeopathic treatments, however, may be affected by certain aromatherapy oils, notably camphor, eucalyptus and peppermint.

Should you or a member of your family ever have major surgery or intense drug treatment for a serious illness, then stress and anxiety are likely to be felt on top of the discomforts of the treatment. During the recovery period, essential oils can help keep the sufferer calm and serene, relieve aches, pains and soreness and build up strength.

While essential oils are on the whole expensive, they do last for quite a long time. Your collection of oils can be built up gradually over a period of time until you have a nicely balanced and varied selection. On a non-therapeutic note, the oils may be used in the home for a wonderful way to enjoy your favourite flower aromas all the year round. An essence burner can create a garden atmosphere in a top-floor flat!

CHAPTER 1

Background to Aromatherapy

A S LONG ago as 4000 BC, the techniques of pressing, boiling and maceration were being used by civilisations in the East to obtain fragrant essences from flowers, leaves, woods, gums and resins. In the process of maceration, for example, the raw material would have been placed in warmed oil or fat and replaced with fresh batches, possibly as many as 15 times. The pomades and aromatic oils thus made were used in unguents (ointments) for anointing kings and holy men and for therapeutic purposes, cosmetics and perfumes.

The Egyptians and Babylonians used lavish amounts of perfumes and perfumed oils. Whilst animal fat was widely used for the basis of unguents, fatty oils were also used, extracted by cold-pressing olives and the seeds of sesame, flax and the castor oil plant. Trade routes were established, for there was a lucrative market in spices, perfumes and incense.

Priests are considered to have been the first retailers of aromatics, dispensing them for perfume as well as for healing purposes. There was no distinction between holy perfumes and household perfumes. Some of the ingredients used then are still used today: frankincense, myrrh, galbanum (gum resins), cedarwood, sandalwood, cypress wood, lavender, camomile, marjoram, oregano, thyme, cinnamon, coriander, clove, roses, lilies, cornflower, jasmine and orange blossom.

The ancient Greeks and Romans also loved scented oils, unguents and pomades. These were so popular in the Roman Empire that quite a flourishing industry was set up. The rose was highly prized and used a great deal in perfumery, medicine and even in food. Roses were tossed at the feet of home-coming Roman conquering armies, and handmaidens strewed rose petals at feasts. In Nero's palace, on special occasions, rooms were carpeted several inches deep in rose petals. The infamous Caligula believed in the therapeutic properties of aromatic baths to restore his body, exhausted by sexual excesses. Julius Caesar, however, did not think much of the highly perfumed Roman males – he preferred them to smell of garlic!

After the fall of the Roman Empire, the use of perfumes and aromatics declined. But during the Middle Ages, the Arabian scientist, physician and philosopher Avicenna discovered (or perhaps rediscovered) the process of distillation for the extraction of rose oil and other plant essences. In fact, his method was to be the basis of our modern distillation processes. Arabian perfumes soon became famous. The Crusaders brought back aromatics from the East to Europe, and before long a perfume industry developed there.

Down the centuries, mankind has relied mainly on plants for medicines. During the nineteenth and twentieth centuries, the science of chemistry developed enormously. Drugs began to be created, and largely supplanted the old herbal medicines – though many modern drugs are still derived from plant sources (for example digitalis, from foxglove).

During the last 200 years, technological advance in the production of essential oils has been considerable, as well as research into their chemistry. The term 'aromatherapy' was coined in 1937 by a French chemist, R-M Gattefossé. He had accidentally discovered the effectiveness of lavender oil on burns while working in a perfumery laboratory. In a small explosion he burned his hand and plunged it into the nearest liquid, which happened to be a bowl of lavender oil. The hand healed very quickly, with hardly a scar.

Subsequently, after researching into the beneficial properties of other essential oils, Gattefossé wrote: 'Doctors and chemists will be surprised at the range of odiferous substances which may be used medicinally and at the great variety of their chemical functions. Besides the antiseptic and antimicrobial properties of which use is currently made, the essential oils are also antitoxic and antiviral, they have a powerful energising effect and possess an undeniable cicatrising property. In the future their role will be even greater.'

That prophecy was to be fulfilled. A number of researchers and pioneers contributed their efforts. Notable among them was a French physician, Dr Jean Valnet, who was inspired by the work of Gattefossé. He used essential oils as antiseptics in the treatment of wounds in World War Two. He also used the oils to combat tuberculosis, diabetes, cancer and other serious illnesses, claiming many successes. In 1964, Valnet published an important book on the subject, *Aromathérapie*.

Aromatherapy was greatly furthered by Marguerite Maury, an Austrian biochemist and beautician. From 1940 until the time of her death in 1968, she published two books, lectured on the subject throughout Europe, and opened aromatherapy centres in Paris, Switzerland and England. She ran courses giving information on the use of essential oils, with emphasis on their rejuvenating and cosmetic effects. Today we are used to the concept of healing holistically, taking the whole person into account and at all levels.

Very early on, Marguerite Maury realised the importance of prescribing for the individual a mixture of oils that would restore balance, not just on the physical level but on the mental and emotional levels too. She was also the first person to establish the technique of applying essential oils, diluted in vegetable oil, by massage.

Over the last 20 years there has been a tremendous upsurge of interest in the therapeutic uses of essential oils. Today, aromatherapy is accepted as a valued branch of complementary medicine and is still fast-growing in popularity.

How Essential Oils Are Obtained

All essential oils are volatile and it is this property, rapid evaporation, that enables us to smell them as the aroma given off is inhaled into our nostriles. Another characteristic of essential oils is that they are not heavy and greasy but generally have quite a watery consistency, though the viscosity does vary from type to type. The thicker ones include sandalwood and patchouli, but even these do not have the greasy texture of the vegetable oils extracted from seeds or nuts, such as sunflower, sesame and coconut.

Oils have a lower density than water – they float on top of it. Essential oils are insoluble in water but they will dissolve in alcohol and other organic liquids, and also in fats, waxes and other oils.

Distillation

Most essential oils are obtained by distillation. The plant material, whatever it happens to be, is placed in a container and either boiled in water or subjected to steam under pressure. The heat causes the oil globules in the material to burst open. The released essence in the form of vapour, together with steam, then passes through a condenser where water cooling takes place. Here the vapours turn back into liquids which are collected in a flask. The essential oil floats on top of the condensed water and is therefore easily separated.

Solvent extraction

The strong heat and pressure used in the distillation process just described would damage the oil of some flowers, notably rose, jasmine and orange blossom. In these cases different methods are used, for example solvent extraction. The essential oil dissolves in the solvent liquid as it flows slowly over the petals.

The solvent is then distilled off at a low temperature. The product, which still contains some waxes, is a semi-solid known as a 'concrete'. When this is shaken in alcohol, the waxes are removed, leaving a high quality flower oil (an 'absolute'). In the past, the solvents used in this method of extraction would have been liquids such as alcohols, petroleum and ether. Today, liquid butane and carbon dioxide are used, producing very high quality oils.

Enfleurage

The oldest method of extracting essential oils is called 'enfleurage', in which the flower essence is absorbed by fat. Sheets of glass are coated with fat, lard for example, over which fresh flowers are sprinkled. The coated glass is then stacked in tiers for many days, during which time the essences are absorbed by the fat. As the flowers deteriorate, they are removed and replaced by new ones. Finally saturation point is reached, when the fat can absorb no more essence, and the fat is then collected. The essence-infused fat (now called a 'pomade') is shaken in alcohol for many hours to separate the essence from the fat. An alternative though similar method uses sheets of muslin stretched over wooden frames and soaked in olive oil. Both these traditional methods, which have been used in the perfume industry, produce very high-quality oils. However, they are time-consuming and the product is therefore very expensive.

Enfleurage is no longer used commercially except to produce oil of tuberose, which is worth its weight in gold. The world's total annual production of tuberose oil is only about 15 kilograms. Cultivated in France and Morocco, the blossoms are hand-picked, wrapped in damp cloths and extracted with lard as outlined above. Tuberose, as far as I'm aware, is not used for aromatherapy – heaven forbid at the price! It is only used in the most expensive perfumes.

Absolutes

The high-quality oils that are the end-product of solvent extraction or enfleurage are termed 'absolutes'. Strictly speaking, only the oils extracted by distillation should be called essential oils. From the point of view of aromatherapy, there is a difference between absolutes and oils obtained by distillation. The former have a stronger perfume and a greater therapeutic power and hence should be used in lower concentrations. Also, they have a thicker consistency and tend to be coloured.

Expression method

The aromatic oils of citrus fruits can be obtained simply by the application of pressure – a method known as 'expression'. Originally the rind of the fruit was squeezed by hand into a sponge to collect the oil. Although the best quality citrus oils are still extracted by hand, machinery is more often used today. The peel is ruptured and the 'cold-pressed' grades of orange, lemon, bergamot, mandarin, grapefruit and lime oils are obtained. Lime oil can also be distilled but the aroma produced in this instance is different.

Because the demand for citrus oils has increased, fruit juice manufacturers have been producing cheaper citrus oils as side products. After the fruit is separated from the pith, it is pulped with the rind to extract the juice. The pulp is then distilled to produce essential oils from the vapour.

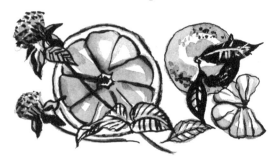

Factors Affecting Composition

The composition of an essential oil can vary quite considerably according to where the plant is grown. Basil, a plant belonging to the *Labiatae* family, produces an oil containing an organic compound called methyl chavicol. The proportion of this substance in basil grown in the Comoro Islands is 80 per cent, whereas basil from Egypt (sometimes called French basil) yields approximately 25 per cent.

Other factors causing variations in the chemical character of specific oils are the particular strain or variety of plant used, the climate in which the plant is grown, the method of agriculture (notably the use or not of pesticides and chemical fertilisers), the soil type and altitude. For example, lavender grown at high altitude produces an oil with a higher ester (linalyl acetate) content, giving it a higher quality aroma.

Natural Versus Synthetic

Think of everything in your home that has a flavour or scent: bottles of perfume and toilet water, soap, shampoo, talcum powder, bath salts, lemon-scented washing-up liquid, fabric conditioner, floor polish – the list is endless. These products all contain aromatic substances, some of which may be essential oils. Some ingredients, though, will be synthetic, that is, produced in a factory and not by a plant.

Let us consider modern perfumes. These generally contain only about 15 per cent natural ingredients, because of the high cost. Very expensive perfumes are likely to contain natural rose oil, but even then the quantity present would only be in the region of one per cent.

Many aromatic substances in commercial use are man-made and rightly so. After all, who needs pure unadulterated essence of pine in a floor-cleaning liquid? Essential oils for use in therapy, however, must be of the finest quality. They should contain neither additives nor chemical extenders as these can damage delicate tissues and, furthermore, are likely to be absorbed by the skin and into the body where harm can be done.

Most plant essences have an extremely complex chemical make-up. They consist of a number of different organic compounds, that is they all contain the element carbon, together with other elements (mainly hydrogen and oxygen). The most common groups of compounds in essential oils are the terpenes, camphenes, derivatives of the phenols and benzene, alcohols, aldehydes and esters, geraniol and linalool. But plant chemistry is for the boffins; we don't need to wrestle with it in order to practise aromatherapy at home.

Chemists are able to analyse the various constituents of a particular oil and combine the separate ingredients in the correct proportions to produce that oil artificially – this can be cheaper than extracting the natural oil. Consider natural rose oil, for example. Perfume chemists know that it contains about 500 substances (the majority of which are present in minute proportions). However, they are getting close to being able to recreate a rose oil that smells just like the natural kind. Whilst reconstituted oils have a place in the perfume industry, their therapeutic potency is usually found to be inferior to that of the natural oils. Why is this so?

There is something about the way natural oils are constructed that chemists have not been able to discover. They cannot reproduce them properly by artificial means – only nature can do that, through the vital energy, the dynamic forces found in living things. Perhaps these same forces have something to do with the healing power of the plant and its essences.

CHAPTER 2

How Aromatherapy Heals

FROM the very earliest times, people have been making use of the beneficial and curative effects of plants. For primitive human beings, finding out which plants have healing properties may have been, initially, a matter of trial and error; perhaps instinct played a part. Once gained, the knowledge would have been passed on, first verbally and then, eventually, in written records.

Hundreds of years ago the first herbals – books about herbs – were written. The medicines described in them were mainly aqueous extractions. These were made either by pouring water over the herb and steeping it, or by simmering and then straining it before drinking. Poultices were the hot application of the herb itself. Ointments would be made by placing the herb in lard until it was saturated with the properties of the herb, then the fat would be melted and run off into jars to cool.

Today, a large number of people are turning to herbal therapy as a more natural, safe form of treatment for their ailments than pharmaceuticals. Unlike our forebears, however, who would have gathered fresh herbs to make infusions and decoctions – usually nasty-tasting – we now tend to purchase packaged pills that are quick and easy to swallow. One can also purchase ready-made tinctures, lotions and ointments for external use.

Active Principles and Properties

Medicinal plants contain active principles, that is compounds that act upon the organism. Some of these compounds have been isolated and are used in modern medicines and drugs, for example atropine from deadly nightshade (*Atropa bella-donna*). Of course many of the medicinal plants are extremely poisonous, as in this example, and are not for use in the home. The fact that a substance comes from a plant does not mean it has no dangerous side effects. There are essential oils, too, which if used in large amounts, and/or too frequently, can do serious harm (see pages 55–6).

The properties of specific medicines are divided into categories according to their physiological effects. For example, a certain medicine or preparation may be described as analgesic (pain-relieving), or carminative (expels wind) and so on. Specific essential oils can be classified in the same way.

Properties of some popular essential oils

ANALGESIC
Pain relieving: bergamot, black pepper, cajeput, camomile, coriander, ginger, lavender, niaouli, peppermint, rosemary, Spanish sage, tea-tree.

ANTIDEPRESSANT
Helps to lift depression: basil (Egyptian), bergamot, camomile, citronella, clary sage, geranium, jasmine, lavandin, lavender, lemongrass, melissa, neroli, orange, patchouli, rose, sandalwood, ylang ylang.

ANTIFUNGAL
See Fungicidal (page 22).

ANTI-INFLAMMATORY
Reduces inflammation: benzoin, cajeput, camomile, coriander, lavandin, lavender, myrrh, orange, peppermint, rose, Spanish sage.

ANTISEPTIC
Kills micro-organisms. Most essential oils are antiseptic to a degree. The following are markedly antiseptic: basil, benzoin, bergamot, black pepper, citronella, dill, eucalyptus, ginger, juniper berry, lavandin, lavender, lemon, lemongrass, mandarin, myrrh, niaouli, orange (sweet), pine, rosemary, sandalwood, Spanish sage, tangerine, tea-tree, thyme, vetiver.

ANTISPASMODIC
Relieves muscle spasm/cramp: basil, black pepper, cajeput, camomile, clary sage, coriander, dill, eucalyptus, fennel, ginger, juniper berry, lavender, mandarin, marjoram, niaouli, orange (sweet), rose, rosemary, Spanish sage, tangerine, thyme, vetiver.

APHRODISIAC
Reputed to increase sexual desire: clary sage, fennel, jasmine, neroli, patchouli, rose, rosemary, sandalwood, ylang ylang.

ASTRINGENT
Contracts tissues and reduces the flow of secretions and discharges: cedarwood, cypress, frankincense, geranium, lemon, lemongrass, patchouli, rose, sage, sandalwood.

CARMINATIVE
Relieves flatulence: camomile, cardamom, clove, fennel, ginger, peppermint, spearmint.

CICATRISANT
Stimulating the formation of scar tissue: frankincense, lavender, neroli, rose, sandalwood.

DEODORANT
Combats body odour: citronella, cypress, eucalyptus, lavender, lemongrass, pine, rosemary, tea-tree.

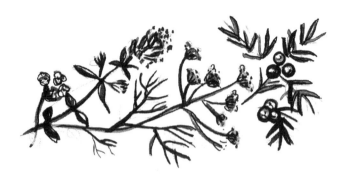

DIURETIC
Promotes the flow of urine: cedarwood, cypress, dill, fennel, geranium, grapefruit, juniper berry, lavender, lemon, mandarin, patchouli, pine, Spanish sage, tangerine, thyme.

EMMENAGOGUE
Induces or stimulates the menstrual flow: basil (Egyptian), camomile, citronella, clary sage, dill, fennel, hyssop, juniper berry, lavandin, lavender, marjoram, myrrh, rose, rosemary, Spanish sage, thyme, vetiver.

EXPECTORANT
Facilitates the break-up of catarrh: basil (Egyptian), benzoin, bergamot, black pepper, cedarwood, eucalyptus, fennel, ginger, hyssop, lavandin, lavender, lemon, myrrh, niaouli, pine, sandalwood, Spanish sage, thyme.

FUNGICIDAL
Inhibits the growth of microscopic fungi: benzoin, lemongrass, myrrh, niaouli, orange, thyme, tea-tree.

HEPATIC
Liver tonics: camomile, cardamom, lemon, peppermint, rose.

HYPERTENSIVE
Raises low blood pressure: rosemary.

HYPOTENSIVE
Reduces high blood pressure: geranium, lavender, lemon, melissa, ylang ylang.

IMMUNO-STIMULANT
Stimulates immune system: cajeput, camomile (German), cedarwood (Atlas), cypress, eucalyptus, frankincense, lemongrass, mandarin, neroli, niaouli, petitgrain, pine, rose, sandalwood, tea-tree, thyme. (See cautionary notes, page 50.)

NERVINE
Tonics for nervous disorders: basil (Egyptian), bay, bergamot, camomile, clary sage, cypress, geranium, jasmine, lavender, lemon, mandarin, marjoram, melissa, neroli, orange, patchouli, peppermint, rose, sandalwood, Spanish sage. For nervines with a mainly calming effect, see Sedative.

RUBEFACIENT
Stimulates peripheral blood supply: black pepper, cajeput, coriander, eucalyptus, ginger, juniper berry, pine, rosemary, thyme, vetiver.

SEDATIVE
Nervines that predominantly calm and soothe: benzoin, camomile, clary sage, juniper berry, mandarin, marjoram, myrrh, neroli, orange, sandalwood, tangerine, vetiver, ylang ylang.

STIMULANT
Excites and increases physical or mental function. Circulatory: black pepper, geranium, ginger, rose, rosemary, thyme, vetiver. Mental: basil (Egyptian), eucalyptus, lemon, lemongrass, peppermint, pine, tea-tree, thyme.

TONIC
Strengthens the whole system, increasing a feeling of well-being: basil (Egyptian), frankincense, geranium, lavandin, lemon, lemongrass, melissa, myrrh, orange, rose, sandalwood, Spanish sage, tangerine, thyme, vetiver.

23

What Is Special about Aromatherapy?

How is it that tiny amounts of essential oils, absorbed into the bloodstream and tissues via the skin, can have marked therapeutic benefits, both physically and mentally?

One possible explanation is that some molecules in essential oils act like hormones; these may form a relationship with our own hormones, travelling through the body systems, revitalising and regulating our emotional and physical responses. Essential oils appear also to stimulate the body's defences against infection. Some essences are more effective than others in this respect, for example tea-tree. They appear to work through their power to promote the formation of the white corpuscles in the blood that attack harmful microbes.

It has been found that certain essential oils have an affinity for particular organs of the body, for example lavender with the kidneys, cypress with the ovaries. It would seem that if an organ is sluggish it will selectively absorb a substance that can boost its action just as it would absorb a nutrient. Dr Valnet suggested that geranium, pine, rosemary and sage stimulate the adrenal cortex (an endocrine gland) and alleviate tension caused by stress. Similarly, mint stimulates the pituitary cortex which affects most of the other hormone-producing glands.

Calming effects of essential oils

It is acknowledged that the mind, emotions and physical body interact. Glands, blood vessels, heart, lungs and intestines are regulated by the nervous system which in turn is affected by the state of our mind. Prolonged stress or anxiety can lead to physical disorders. Overstimulation of gastric juices, for example, may give rise to peptic ulcers.

Apart from the tension-relieving effect mentioned above, the mind and emotions may be soothed by essential oils in other ways. For example, an oil may have a direct sedative or stimulating effect on the nerves. In particular, the very perception of a pleasant fragrance can have a soothing, uplifting effect, dispelling depression.

Different odours, nice, nasty or indifferent, affect our moods in various ways. The nerve pathways associated with the sense of smell are in very close proximity to the brain. They connect with a part of the brain known as the limbic system, which is responsible for our feelings and emotions. This is largely why the aromas of essential oils can have such an influence on our moods and feelings. We will pursue the subject of the sense of smell more fully in the next chapter.

When using essential oils, it is apparent that some of them have both a stimulating and a sedative effect. This seems like a contradiction but it is not. If you want to feel calm and relaxed but not drowsy as you need to continue with work, one of the following oils would be a good choice: basil, bergamot, grapefruit, lavender or tangerine. On the other hand, if you want to relax totally to the point of being half asleep, you could choose a sedative oil such as camomile, clary sage, jasmine or vetiver.

How aromatherapy differs from herbal medicine

Although aromatherapy is allied to herbal medicine in that they are both based on substances derived from plants, there are distinct differences. The properties of an extracted plant essence are not likely to be exactly the same as those of a herbal infusion or decoction, albeit from the same kind of plant. The preparation techniques are different, and these have a bearing on the chemical constituents, and therefore the properties, of the end-product. Heat is usually employed both in the production of herbal extracts, that is those used as medicines, and in the extraction of essential oils. Boiling can destroy some ingredients but, on the other hand, some volatile oils need a sustained high temperature to permit extraction.

The very process of distillation can alter the constituents of an oil. A very good case in point is the essential oil of camomile. This contains a blue-violet crystalline substance called azulene. Azulene is not present in the fresh flower but is formed when the oils are distilled. Azulene is a healing agent for skin conditions (see page 77).

There is some evidence that when a known active constituent is present in an essential oil, its properties may be found to be greater than when it has been isolated and used alone for treatment. A possible explanation is that the minor constituents of the oil contribute in a major way to its therapeutic properties (as well as to its colour and odour). To give an example, it has been demonstrated that the essential oil of eucalyptus has greater antiseptic properties than isolated eucalyptol, its principal constituent. An analogy may be made here with vitamins. It is now widely recognised that other substances have to be present with a vitamin for it to be fully utilised in the body. Vitamin C is a good case in point. Its action is helped by the substances known as bioflavonoids, which always accompany the vitamin in foods and are sometimes included in vitamin C tablets.

When isolated, some constituents of essential oils can have an irritant effect on the skin, though when the rest of the constituents of the natural oil are present no skin reaction occurs. An example of this is oil of lemongrass, which contains citral, an aldehyde that will cause a skin reaction if used in isolation. (Some essential oils are actually toxic, and of course these are not used in aromatherapy.)

Many aromatherapists claim that the therapeutic properties of essential oils tend to be greater in combination than when used alone – the components are said to be working 'synergistically'. I am not wholly convinced that this is so, though blending is useful in that one can combine several therapeutic properties in one treatment as well as creating delightful aromas.

Some further aspects of healing

An important part of aromatherapy is massage, which encourages absorption of oils into the skin and stimulates the circulation (see Chapter 8). The caring human touch and the ability to be able to talk about personal problems without fear of criticism can aid the healing process.

A good aromatherapist will take into consideration the whole person and not just the ailing part or symptom. The subject of 'holistic' healing is too deep and involved to be dealt with adequately here, but its basic principles can be mentioned. If you are ill and in pain, a practitioner will treat the symptom first to relieve the discomfort. A holistic practitioner will also, in the longer term, treat the fundamental cause in an effort to prevent the problem recurring. Not only the body but the mind and spirit need to be taken into account. A balance needs to be brought about within the whole self for health, well-being, inner peace and tranquillity. Aromatherapy is an ideal means towards achieving this.

Professional Treatment

Qualified aromatherapists treat clients for a variety of conditions, such as arthritis, circulatory problems, anxiety and depression, muscular stress and strain, migraines, menopausal troubles and rheumatism. The client is treated at a salon, clinic, private practice, or at home by a 'mobile therapist'.

If you consult an aromatherapist, initially you will be asked about your general health, eating and sleeping habits, amount of exercise and medical background. Then the therapist will make up a blend of essential oils for massage. These will be the ones considered right for you as a whole person rather than just your symptoms. Many aromatherapists also use reflexology (treatment of specific ailments by foot massage) before a massage, as this helps pinpoint energy imbalance.

The results of aromatherapy treatment are usually seen after three or four sessions. Weekly or fortnightly sessions may be recommended to begin with, perhaps reducing to once a month. The improvement may be maintained by using the prescribed blend of oils at home. Clients may decide to have treatment once a week indefinitely, if they wish to maintain a permanent state of relaxation and well-being.

The massage relaxes both mind and body, relieving tension and anxiety. Unfortunately, many people wait until something goes wrong before they seek help. When aromatherapy treatments are kept up regularly (at least once a month), all the systems are revitalised. This not only eliminates a good number of everyday problems but, in my opinion, helps to prevent major disease.

One of the benefits of visiting a therapist is the comfort factor. By this I mean the emotional support you get from human touch, and the relationship with a therapist – built on trust. You are able to unburden your problems without fear of criticism or judgement. Being able to talk about your troubles in total confidence is one of the factors that promote health and well-being.

Choosing the Right Therapist

It is very important to consult a fully qualified and fully insured practitioner and personal recommendation is by far the best way to find someone who is experienced. Just having some idea of who you are going to puts any doubts or fears to rest, and makes for a more personalised introduction. Personal recommendation is not always possible, however, so the next step is to make enquiries via an accredited association. Associations keep a register of qualified practitioners who have been trained to the high standards set down in a core curriculum by the AOC (Aromatherapy Organisations Council). The Council have the details of associations and their respective training establishments, and from this information you will be able to find a therapist in your area. To obtain information, contact the Secretary, Aromatherapy Organisations Council, 3 Latymer Close, Braybrooke, Market Harborough, Leics, LE16 8LN; Tel/Fax 01858 434242.

If you decide to contact someone who has advertised, ask the following questions before making an appointment:

- Where did you train?
- How long was the training, and did you gain a diploma?
- Do you belong to an association?
- Do you have public liability insurance?
- Do you take a full medical history as part of the consultation?

If the therapist is reluctant to give you this information, or is unclear with the answers, avoid booking the appointment. The ideal answers are:

- I trained with an AOC approved or affiliated training school.
- The course was in excess of 200 hours, over a one-year period, and yes, I gained a diploma.
- I belong to an accredited association of the AOC.
- I carry public liability and professional indemnity insurance.
- Yes, I take a full initial consultation lasting at least 30 minutes.

Properly trained therapists will not be offended at these questions, so don't feel embarrassed, I am sure that they will be proud of their training and qualifications. Also be sure to confirm the duration and costs of treatment, including consultation, before booking.

CHAPTER 3

The Sense of Smell

WE ARE capable of recognising 4,000 different scents, and a highly sensitive nose might be able to identify as many as 10,000. When somebody is blind and deaf, the enormous potential of the sense of smell compensates for the loss of hearing and sight.

How do we smell something? Here is a very brief summary. Specialised cells in the nasal cavity receive stimuli from the airborne odour particles, olfactory nerves transmit the stimuli to the brain where the signals are passed along the olfactory tract to several brain areas, and nerve cells in the temporal lobes of the cerebrum (part of the fore-brain) interpret the stimuli.

It is worth looking into the process in more detail.

In the upper part of the mucous membrane of the nasal cavities, on each side, is a little patch of receptor cells. Although each of these olfactory membranes is not much larger than a thumbnail, together they contain approximately 20 million receptor cells. Projecting from each cell are eight or more fibrils which identify the scent. Odour molecules reaching the receptor cells stimulate them to send rapid impulses through adjoining nerve fibres.

These nerve fibres from the receptor cells pass through tiny apertures in a wafer-thin section of bone called the cribriform plate which is at the front of the cranial cavity. The nerve fibres run directly into two outlying portions of the brain called the olfactory bulbs. No bigger than match heads, the bulbs are located just behind the bridge of the nose and about 1 cm (½ in) into the head. From this region, sensations are passed along a web of nerve tracts into many parts of the brain.

Most of the nerve pathways associated with smell terminate in the central regions of the brain which are thought to have been the earliest to develop during the course of evolution. These are the parts mostly responsible for our basic emotions and sexual behaviour. There are further connections with the pituitary gland, the master gland of the endocrine system. Some connections, of course, are made with the outer part of the brain (the cortex). This region of the brain developed later on, and is responsible for higher thought processes.

Thoughts and feelings interact with one another. Some scientists go so far as to assert that all our emotions are the result of neurochemicals and hormones released into the bloodstream. Be that as it may, essential oils are widely believed to stimulate or normalise the release of hormones and neurochemicals in the body (massage is also said to bring this about). This explains why aromatherapy brings about a state of well-being.

It has also been claimed that essential oils themselves act like hormones in the body, stimulating glandular secretions. Whether this is so or not, one can at least say that the effect of the essences on the emotions and on the nervous system suggests an influence on the endocrine system. Fennel oil is known to contain a form of the hormone oestrogen. For this reason it is often used to treat menstrual disorders, but it should be avoided in pregnancy.

Some aromas can trigger the release of memories, either pleasant or unpleasant.

Through the effects that certain essential oils have upon our senses they can help us to clarify our thoughts, be more aware of ourselves (and others) and act more positively.

Scientists have begun to unravel the complex hormonal and neurological avenues relating to smell. They now predict that in the future it will be possible to manipulate mood, emotions and behaviour by using the right scents (to some extent, that is what aromatherapists have been doing for some while). A recent report on scientific research into the use of aroma says that, although it sounds like science fiction, aromas were being formulated that could stimulate or calm people. It was also suggested that directors of large companies should give a quick spray of an 'aroma activate' before summoning executives for important board meetings.

Today, some hospitals and surgeries use citrus or woody smells to allay patients' fears. Office workers have also been exposed to specific aromas to increase their alertness (an essence burner on every desk). Computer workers in Japan have been found to perform more efficiently after their working environment was scented with lemon.

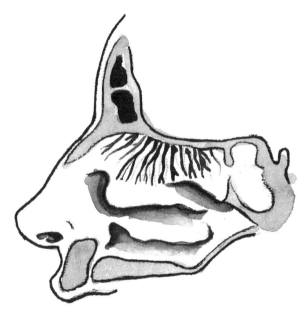

Filaments of the olfactory nerves

Warwick University experts developed an aroma reminiscent of the seaside. It was believed to be a blend of seaweed aroma, woody fragrances and sun lotion. This was used experimentally in the treatment of severe chronic anxiety and agoraphobia (fear of open spaces).

The scientists still have some mysteries to solve relating to the sense of smell. Although they have been able to demonstrate that in the sense of taste – to which smell is closely related – there are four primary flavours (sweet, sour, bitter and salt), they have not been as successful in classifying smells. Some say there are seven basic odours, others say there are 50 or more, and still others maintain that every odour is a primary one.

The Art of Smelling Essential Oils

Most people's sense of smell is underdeveloped and needs to be trained. So, before launching into the practical techniques of aromatherapy, let's begin with some experiments that will enhance your powers of distinguishing aromas.

First of all, obtain at least four essential oils, but no more than six. More than this will confuse your nose and eventually you will not be able to differentiate between the odours. Cedarwood will smell like lavender and lavender like rosemary. (Lemongrass will always smell like lemongrass!)

Next, choose an area away from other strong aromas (kitchens, etc.). The temperature of the room should be warm and it should be free from draughts. Breathe in and out quite quickly through your nose in order to clear the nasal passages.

Write the name of each essential oil you are going to test on coffee filter papers or strips of blotting paper. Test one oil at a time. Dip the end of the strip – about 1cm (½ in) – into the oil. Then hold the paper just under your nose – about 1–2 cm (½–1 in) away – avoiding touching the skin.

When I am conducting a lesson on essences, I ask my

students to write down their impressions of the aroma. As well as describing the quality of the aroma, they record the mental effect it has on them, for example, sedative, stimulating, uplifting, refreshing.

Aromas are usually defined in 'notes'.

Top note	This is the characteristic first impression. Top notes are sharpish, evaporate quickly, and usually last 20–30 minutes.
Middle note	This is classed as the heart or bouquet and fully develops between one and two hours, sometimes longer. It lasts for a day or two.
Base note	The bottom note is the heaviest, gives an aroma its strength and is the last to fade.

These notes sometimes overlap, so you may find a base note that will also show a middle note and a middle note showing a top note.

Try the following experiment. Pour a few drops of different essential oils on to separate pieces of blotting paper and smell them at intervals. Which ones are the first to fade? Does the aroma alter after a time? Oils that have a predominant top note include bergamot, eucalyptus, lemon, tea-tree. Oils with a distinctive base note include frankincense, sandalwood and ylang ylang. Somewhere in the middle you will find camomile, fennel and geranium. These are just a few examples.

The following terms are used to describe the aromas:

BALSAMIC
Warm and sweet with a soft odour of resins.

CAMPHORACEOUS
Clean and medicinal.

HERBACEOUS
Having a distinct odour of herbs or garden plants.

METALLIC
Cold steel, cool and clear.

GREEN
Fresh and grass-like.

SPICY
Having an aroma reminiscent of cinnamon or nutmeg, warm.

WOODY
A warm, leaf-like aroma more than a definite wood tone.

FRUITY
Having an aroma of fruit (apples, pears, etc.).

FLORAL
Usually a sweet aroma, smelling of flowers.

SWEET
An aroma like vanilla, peach or jam.

CITRUS
Fresh tangy orange, lemon or lime tones.

Try describing a few essential oils using the above terms. Record the aroma after 15 minutes, 30 minutes, two hours, one day, one week. The examples below will serve as a guide:

GERANIUM

Top note	Powerful, sweet, honey-like, rosy odour with minty fresh undertones.
Middle note	Still minty – rose tone deepens.
Base note	Still a trace of mintiness – rose tone is slightly peppery and metallic.

EUCALYPTUS

Top note   Pungent, refreshing, camphoraceous, head-clearing.

Middle note   Slightly woody tone.

Base note   Non-existent.

ROSE ABSOLUTE

Top note   Rich and rosy, like tea with honey, soft and floral.

Middle note   Richer honey tones, still rosy.

Base note   Still rosy in character – honey tone not as sweet.

YLANG YLANG

Top note   Warm, floral, slightly medicinal – the better-quality oil is very like jasmine.

Middle note   Floral tone develops – warmer.

Base note   More like jasmine – still rich and floral.

Make Your Own Blends

Having trained your nose, you should find no difficulty blending oils together to achieve really satisfying aromas. You will find out which oils tend to be overpowering in a blend and are best used in tiny amounts. In a good blend the components will complement each other. For example, try sharp, sweet oils such as citrus (lemon, mandarin, sweet orange, grapefruit) with warm, spicy ones such as ginger, coriander, cardamom. The soft woody tone of sandalwood blends well with a floral type, such as geranium, rose or ylang ylang.

CHAPTER 4

Buying and Storing Your Oils

MOST essential oils will remain effective for up to two years, provided they are kept in suitable containers. They are usually supplied in dark glass bottles – amber, dark green or blue. If you change the container, make sure you label it clearly. When mixing blends, keep them in similar glass bottles, which you can buy from a chemist. Plastic bottles cannot be used as containers for more than eight weeks as the oils will deteriorate.

The vegetable oils used as a base for essential oils will not hold the aroma or properties of the essence for very long; without preservatives the vegetable oil will oxidise, resulting in loss of effectiveness. For this reason, I suggest making up no more than 100 ml at any one time.

Store your oils in a cool place out of direct sunlight and away from naked flames. As essential oils are volatile, make sure the bottle top is always properly secured.

Keep essential oils away from children. Do not keep them in any bottle or location where they could be mistaken for medicines or drinks.

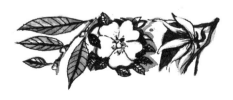

Purchasing Essential Oils

It is advisable to find a reputable supplier because descriptions in sales literature cannot always be relied upon. If you have any difficulty, I can vouch for the purity and quality of the oils marketed by the mail order companies whose details are given on page 218.

By means of highly sensitive chemical tests – gas chromatography – it is possible for companies to find out whether the oils sent to them by suppliers are indeed unadulterated and of a purity essential for use in aromatherapy. The colour of particular oils may vary a little from time to time. But if you find that all the essential oils you have purchased are colourless, there is a problem somewhere!

Availability and price of essential oils

Generally speaking, the cost of a particular oil is higher the lower the yield per kilo of plant material used in its production. There are exceptions, however. Lavender yields quite a low percentage of essential oil per load (approximately 1.6 per cent) but the oil is relatively inexpensive (about £4.50 per 10 ml bottle at the time of writing). This is because lavender is widely cultivated; literally fields and fields of it are grown in many countries of the world, and therefore it is available in large quantities. Also, lavender doesn't need fertilisers or pesticides (see page 39).

Frankincense and myrrh yield quite a large percentage of oil from the gum resin but they are quite expensive in comparison with lavender (about £13.00 per 10 ml bottle). The trees grow wild and crops are comparatively scarce. Sandalwood, again fairly pricey, is not considered oil-producing until the trees are 25–30 years old.

Details of the most popular and useful essential oils are given in Chapter 7.

Organically grown oils

The fashion now is for 'organic' oils. All living plants are organic, of course. The usual definition of 'organically grown' is that the plants are produced in conformity with the strict guidelines set down by the Soil Association. It takes five years or more for soil to become free of chemicals; therefore if plants are not sprayed with chemicals but grown in unclean soil they are not strictly 'organic'. If you see any product sold as 'organic' that does not carry the Soil Association's symbol, the seller should be challenged.

Overseas, producers and sellers of organically grown produce come under the umbrella of the International Federation of Organic Agricultural Movement (IFOAM). Eventually EU regulations will make it illegal to sell products as organically grown unless they carry the EU organic symbol or that of the designated governmental body which in the United Kingdom is the Soil Association.

Meanwhile, certain companies are making extraordinary claims in this field. At present there are very few organically grown essential oils on the market, and since they are only available in very small quantities they command a high price. Lavender is one of the exceptions. The plant produces its own insecticide, so it doesn't need to be sprayed with chemicals. It will also grow on poor soils and therefore doesn't require the application of fertilisers. Lavender oil is therefore naturally organic.

'Pure' (and 'pure organic') oils

An essential oil described as 'pure' should not have been mixed or diluted with any other substance. Ideally it should be free from tainting or polluting matter. Nevertheless, it would not be quite accurate to state that it is 100 per cent pure because almost certainly there will be impurities present, such as traces of substances from the soil in which the plant grew and possibly also air pollutants.

Ideally, all essential oils for use in aromatherapy should be organically grown and distilled with care. Growers and producers are likely to become increasingly more aware of this need as the popularity of aromatherapy grows.

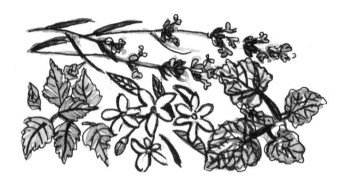

'Natural' oils

This description means existing in or produced by nature. Strictly speaking, only those essential oils obtained from plants grown in the wild can be called 'natural'. But the plants mainly used nowadays in the production of essential oils are specially cultivated for the purpose. They are propagated by taking cuttings and grafting, which again is not 'natural'.

'True' oils

This word is being used to define essential oils. It means factually accurate, not false, fictional or illusory. But what does the retailer mean by 'true'? True to botanical source, purity and nature? Or true, it was man-made in a laboratory? 'True' certainly sounds nice, and reputable companies will use this adjective for all the right reasons. The problem is, relatively unknown companies with no established credentials are describing their wares as 'pure and natural true organic oils'!

In the early days, companies selling essential oils were all guilty of labelling oils as 100 per cent pure/natural/unadulterated. Now I believe the companies with integrity have dropped the hype and are relying on their reputation, knowledge and understanding of essential oils; they use expressions such as top- or high-quality, simply implying general excellence.

Watch out for adulteration

So-called 'nature identicals' are substances produced chemically for the perfume industry. These can be used to adulterate or even 'make' essential oils for the unsuspecting supplier. Another method of adulteration is to extend or 'cut', either with a chemical substance or with terpenes removed from other essential oils. You have to know, and trust, your supplier very well or send your oils away for analysis (hardly practical).

The greatest problem is the supplier who knows little about essential oils. I have been astounded at the blatant adulteration of essential oils in some retail outlets. I remember going into a craft shop recently where, among the pot pourri, scented candles and suchlike, there was a display of '100 per cent pure essential oils for aromatherapy'. My curiosity got the better of me and I started testing them. They were dreadful, obviously not from any natural botanical source. The viscosity was wrong and my nose smelt a rat (figuratively, of course). One of the first signs that told me they were not pure was the price. Sandalwood, jasmine and neroli were all priced at £2.95 for 25 ml. When I challenged the shopkeepers, a young couple, they assured me that the oils were indeed 100 per cent pure. I asked them how they could be sure and whether they knew anything about aromatherapy. They both looked rather shocked and sheepish, saying their supplier had told them the oils were pure.

'Aromatherapy oils'

The public can be misled by products described as 'aromatherapy oils'. These are essential oils that have been put into a vegetable or mineral oil. It is not an adulteration if the literature on the bottle states clearly that it is a blended oil ready for application. If, on the other hand, it is sold as essential oil, it would be classified as adulterated.

This can be an excellent way of buying the more expensive oils (rose, neroli and jasmine), provided of course the essential oils are genuine. Market intelligence on suppliers is not easy to come by. Ask questions and study the literature of the seller. Use your intuition and start to train your nose. If a company appears to be selling oils all at the same price or too cheaply, buyer beware!

Signs to look for

If you have tried the exercises for training your nose (pages 33–6), you will easily be able to carry out the following test. Drop a little of the suspicious oil on to a piece of blotting paper. If the aroma disappears too quickly, adulteration is likely – probably with alcohol.

Now test the texture. If it is oily and spreads either on paper or on your skin, it has had an oil of vegetable origin added to it. Oils that are extended leave an oily residue.

We know that essential oils have a shelf life and are usually stored in amber or dark brown bottles. If an oil is sold in a clear glass bottle, be suspicious.

Labelling of Essential Oils

The labelling of essential oils comes under the scrutiny of the MCA (Medicines Control Agency) and the ATC (Aromatherapy Trades Council). The two organisations are currently working together to regulate the information given out by companies who sell essential oils. The ATC, however, can only monitor and represent its particular membership and does not have any authority over companies outside its association. The MCA enforces the legislation regarding the claiming of cures for medical conditions: for example, a bottle of marjoram cannot be labelled as a cure or remedy for arthritis, as this is considered to be a medical condition; this also applies to blended massage oils and lotions. The MCA also classes headaches, migraine, stress and anxiety as medical conditions. However, I was amused to find out several years ago that the symptoms of menopause were not considered to be medical conditions; I wonder, could the department have been run by men?

A few years ago, the EU powers that be in Brussels wanted to restore the licensing of all herbal products. This caused some anxiety in the aromatherapy profession, as it was thought the legislation would affect the sale of essential oils, but fortunately the bill was overturned and things are, at present, as they were. However, Brussels seems intent on trying to interfere in the complementary medicine profession, so who knows what lies in store for all of us.

What to look for

The label naming the oil will either say 'Oil of Lavender' or 'Lavender Oil' and should also state that it is a pure essential oil. You may also find the botanical name has been added. The most popular size bottle sold is 10 ml which is only a couple of centimetres high; therefore the labels are small, and the amount of information which can be printed is very limited. The information on a label is important, as leaflets given out with the product can be lost, or not read fully on purchase. It is very important that the main warnings such as 'Do not take internally', 'Dilute before use', 'Keep oils away from children', should be clearly visible.

Anything labelled as an 'aromatherapy oil' should state that it is pure essential oil blended in a particular base oil. If the product is being sold as a single essential oil, it is helpful to know the dilution rate.

A good-quality pure essential oil should have a strong and, more importantly, a lasting aroma. If the aroma dies very quickly, it means the product is not high quality. If you want more information on the essential oils you are buying, contact the company direct. They should be able to give you the answers in a confident and reassuring manner; if they do not, think again.

Containers

The kind of containers that are most useful for making and storing your favourite recipes should be made of glass or polyplastics. To keep undiluted essential oil formulas, use amber or dark blue glass bottles, of 10 ml, 25 ml or 50 ml.

Citrus oils keep longer and fresher if kept in the fridge; if made into a massage oil, remember to take the bottle out at least a half hour before use, or the cold will give you a shock.

You can warm massage oils by standing the bottle in a bowl of hot water – warmed massage oil is very, very soothing.

Other containers for home-made formulas of oils, creams or lotions need not be larger than 50–100 ml, as this quantity will last for some time. Always use clean and sterile containers, as any previous content, if not fully removed, will spoil your blend. If you are making up larger quantities of oil to use for the whole family, then a bottle of 250 ml will be sufficient.

Bottles, jars and plastic bottles are usually available from mail order suppliers (see pages 218–9), chemists or cash and carry beauty suppliers, or you might like to re-use empty cold cream pots, bubble bath and shampoo bottles. To clean them thoroughly, pop them in the dishwasher when there is a space, making sure they are made of robust plastic. Label the bottles and jars clearly, and keep them away from young children.

Bases

Vegetable oils are used in aromatherapy massage blends. They serve to dilute the essential oils, which are too strong to be applied direct to the skin. The base oil also acts as a lubricant for the hands during massage.

If you dislike the feel of oil on your skin, an alternative is to use a white lotion base. Several mail order companies supply lotion bases, including the ones named on pages 218–9.

Purchasing base oils

When choosing base oils for your massage blends, my advice again is to buy only top quality even though it costs more. The best vegetable oils are extra virgin, that is cold-pressed from the first pressing. In later extractions, heat and solvents are used.

Avoid mineral oils as bases as they have little penetrating power. They stay on the surface of the skin and impede the absorption of essential oils. Furthermore, mineral oils have a drying effect with prolonged use. Baby oil, incidentally, is sometimes mineral-based and may contain synthetic perfumes.

Choosing your base

There are a number of vegetable oils widely used as bases. They all have their own characteristics and special uses. It is worth remembering that some vegetable oils are nourishing for dry and ageing skin, and several contain useful amounts of minerals and vitamins. Vitamin E oil can be added to any base oil to improve dry skin.

The lighter oils are the best all-purpose carriers. Some of the vegetable oils that are rich in vitamin E are also rather thick and sticky; they need to be blended with less viscous oils (at 10–20 per cent). Any oil you wish to use that is expensive or has a strong odour can be blended with other oils.

Any oil may cause an allergic reaction in certain people with highly sensitive skins. This very rarely happens but for safety's sake you should do a patch test first (see page 54) before making up your massage blend.

The following vegetable oils are among those used by aromatherapists:

ALMOND (SWEET)
My favourite. A light but nourishing oil suited to most skin types and soothing to any irritations. It contains vitamin E so keeps very well.

APRICOT KERNEL
Light texture, a good source of vitamins and minerals, but expensive and not easily obtainable.

ARACHIS
See Peanut (page 48).

AVOCADO
Heavy, rich in vitamins and readily absorbed. Specially good for dry or mature skins. It is best blended with a lighter oil.

COCONUT
The oil is fractionated, which means that during the pressing process it is heated and a fraction – the lighter oil – is extracted, leaving heavy fatty acids and wax behind. The resulting light-textured oil is becoming very popular, being non-greasy, easily absorbed and nourishing. Suitable for all skin types.

CORN
Light texture, nourishing (contains vitamins and minerals). Inexpensive and suitable for all skin types.

GRAPESEED
Light texture, odourless, easily absorbed. For all skin types, especially oily ones.

HAZELNUT
Light texture, good penetrative power, contains vitamins and minerals. For all skin types, especially oily ones.

JOJOBA
Really fine-textured, but best blended with a lighter oil. Good for facial blends and skin troubles such as acne, eczema, psoriasis. Rich in vitamin E. Stays fresh for longer than most oils – add it to massage oils to extend their life.

OLIVE
Sticky, not a good lubricant, and has a strong odour. But this oil has healing properties, for example it is good for dry or sore skin. Best when added to other oils. Readily available.

PEACH KERNEL
Light texture, contains useful nutrients, expensive. It is sometimes sold mixed with apricot-kernel oil (both are getting scarce).

PEANUT

Also known as arachis oil. Rich in vitamins and minerals. Suitable for use on its own. Eases rheumatism of the joints.

SAFFLOWER

Light texture, good penetrative power, quite a good source of minerals and vitamins, cheap and readily available. For all skin types.

SESAME

Heavy texture, best added to other oils. The toasted variety is unsuitable, having a strong odour. The unrefined oil is a good source of vitamin E. This oil is reputed to help skin ailments and rheumatism.

SOYA

Light-textured, inexpensive, but unless of good quality quickly turns rancid. It is nourishing, quickly absorbed and suitable for all skin types.

SUNFLOWER

Light-textured, a source of minerals and vitamins, inexpensive. For all skin types.

VITAMIN E

Improves dry and mature skins and helps heal scars. Blend with other oils.

WHEATGERM

Dark with a pronounced odour, heavy and sticky, not a good lubricant, and expensive. Some people are allergic to wheatgerm. On the positive side, the oil is a rich source of vitamin E (improves dry skin, is good for healing burns and helps prevent scar tissue). Vitamin E is an anti-oxidant – a few drops added to your massage oils will prolong their shelf life.

CHAPTER 5

Cautionary Notes

*T*HIS is a short chapter but a very important one. Before you use essential oils on yourself, your family or friends it is necessary to know when to exercise caution. But, provided you use common sense and take heed of the warnings given, essential oils are a very safe treatment for all kinds of conditions.

Special Cases

Babies and young children have delicate skin, so use only the oils recommended as particularly gentle and suitable for them (see pages 138–40).

During pregnancy, only certain oils are considered safe (see pages 129–30). Halve the amounts you would normally use. Avoid all others.

Epileptics or **anyone with brain damage** should not be given aniseed, star anise, camphor, fennel, hyssop, rosemary or sage.

There are oils that can be specially recommended for the **elderly,** see Chapter 12.

Asthmatics may be affected by certain essential oils; either consult a professional aromatherapist or use the recommended oils at low dosage.

Physically or mentally handicapped people of any age may be given aromatherapy treatment. At first, though, reduce the amount of essential oils in any given formula to about a half. You will soon get to know how the person responds and can either increase or decrease amounts by a few drops if necessary.

Inhalation of essential oils can calm a troubled, perplexed mind, making it an ideal form of treatment for the handicapped. Consider arranging for the person to receive regular treatment from a professional aromatherapist. Nowadays therapists are using their skills with essential oils to improve communication and co-operation in areas that have proved difficult before. When the art of massage is used, words are not necessary; the caring touch is a better way of breaking down communication barriers.

Care should be taken if you are on **hormone replacement therapy (HRT)**: some essential oils have similar properties to oestrogen, for example fennel and coriander, and these should be avoided if you are on oestrogen supplements or patches. Clary sage and Spanish sage should only be used in low dosage if on hormone replacement, as they might upset the balance. If you are unsure, consult a qualified aromatherapist.

Avoid the use of particular essential oils if you have undergone a **liver transplant operation,** or have had **liver disease** such as auto immune hepatitis or primary biliary cirrhosis. The oils to avoid are classed as immuno-stimulants (stimulating to the immune system) and would be contra-indicated if you are on immunosuppressants, medication given to suppress the action of rejection by antibodies. Immuno-stimulants relating to the oils contained in this book are cajeput, camomile (German), cedarwood (Atlas), cypress, eucalyptus, frankincense, lemongrass, mandarin, neroli, niaouli, petitgrain, pine, rose, sandalwood, tea-tree and thyme. This information applies to any transplant treated with immunosuppressants.

Cancer treatment – radiotherapy and chemotherapy: if you would like to have aromatherapy massage whilst undergoing treatment for cancer, or want to give massage to a cancer sufferer, you must take the following precautions. Always obtain clearance from the medical practitioner in charge of your case. The site and type of cancer must be noted and whether the cancer has secondaries, or if the lymph nodes are affected. Ideally the therapist should have been trained in the treatment of cancer conditions. Do not treat areas such as the site of the cancer, and the site of any treatment such as radiotherapy; avoid tumours, open wounds, inflammation, bruising or scar tissue. Stop treatment if acute pain is present. Aromatherapy treatments should not be given directly prior or immediately after chemo- or radiotherapy. If the patient and doctor agree, treatment might be beneficial midway between treatments. Chemotherapy and radiotherapy can cause the skin to become very sensitive, and there is also the danger of thrombosis, phlebitis and bruising due to the effects on the blood platelets, and so massage must be carried out only if these cautions have been thoroughly checked and discussed. If massage is not advisable, essential oils can be used with compresses, or gentle stroking, or holding of the hands or face for comfort. Caution must always be exercised and the dosage of blends must be very weak. Using an essence burner to ease anxiety is very helpful.

Clinical depression is a medical condition and different from the general feeling of being depressed, fed up, low in salts. Clinical depression is usually caused by chemical disturbances in the brain resulting in an imbalance of moods. It may be triggered by extreme stress, shock, psychological problems and genetic predisposition and it is a serious condition mainly treated by drugs and therapy. Clinical depression can be helped by aromatherapy, but should not be used in place of prescribed medication, unless under supervision by a medical practitioner. Avoid the use of marjoram, as it can cause a stupefying effect and might be contra-indicated to tranquillisers.

If you are suffering from any serious illness, mental condition or skin condition that requires you to be on **steroids** or **tranquillisers,** always inform your doctor if you intend to consult a therapist or use home treatment. Nowadays, many doctors are in favour of aromatherapy and will be supportive of such a suggestion.

First Aid Action

If you have an adverse skin reaction to any essential oil, remove the oil immediately with soap and warm water. If possible, shower the oils off, and soap several times; it is not advisable to soak in the bath, as this will encourage the oils to penetrate further. If irritation persists, seek medical advice.

If your child or a member of your family accidentally swallows neat essential oils, the following emergency procedure should be followed. *Do not under any circumstances induce vomiting,* as this may damage the delicate tissue of the digestive tract and possibly cause irritation to the air passages. Administer a glass of semi-skimmed or diluted full-fat milk immediately. Next, try to establish how much oil was ingested. If the amount swallowed by a child is only one or two drops, there is no need to rush them off to hospital, unless they show signs of trauma. The glass of milk, followed by plenty of fluids such as water or fruit juice should be sufficient; however, if after taking the fluids the child shows signs of sickness, seek medical advice. If the amount was in the region of a teaspoon or more, administer milk or tepid water and call the emergency services. Essential oils are usually sold in bottles with integral droppers and therefore large amounts would be difficult for a child to swallow; also the taste is so horrible, that one would hope this would deter the child from wanting to swallow much, but the danger of a large dose cannot be ruled out.

The risk of fatality is rare, but would depend on the essential oil ingested; for example 1–2 ml of basil or camphor might well cause serious poisoning. If the same dosage of citrus oils were swallowed, the major risk would be to the digestive tract lining and should be treated with the same emergency treatment. If you suspect essential oil poisoning some of the symptoms are: nausea, vomiting, convulsions, colic, dizziness, muscle cramps, diarrhoea, sweating, listlessness and breathing difficulties. These symptoms would only occur in extreme cases where a child had ingested a large dose of a hazardous oil, and it had not been detected for some time. Do not be alarmed by this information, however, as cases of poisoning by the ingestion of essential oils are very rare, but do be aware that the danger exists and information on emergency procedures must be available.

Oil may get into the eyes if a child is inquisitive and tries to look into the dropper by holding the bottle over the face. Flush the eye with tepid to warm water for at least ten minutes. *Do not use carrier oil,* as this will dissolve the essential oil which might then be absorbed into the eye where it could damage delicate eye tissue; this would also impair medical treatment. When you have flushed the eye, seek medical advice.

Frequency of Use

I would advise taking a break from essential oils of at least 24 hours in any one week. But if you want to use them in the bath or in massage oils every day, drink extra water (this aids elimination of toxins). Restrict yourself to the mildest oils and reduce the recommended amounts by half.

In particular heed the cautions in Chapter 7 where you are exhorted to use certain oils in moderation – that means a maximum of three to four drops once or twice a week.

For therapy, it should not be necessary to use essential oils every day unless treating specific areas, such as painful joints or skin problems. As symptoms improve, the oils/lotions will be needed less often. Aromatherapy baths can be taken two or three times a week until the condition has significantly diminished, and then once or twice a week for maintenance.

Essence burners can be used on a daily basis because the oils are not in direct contact with the skin and are sufficiently diffused – it is still a good idea to drink extra water.

As a general rule, it is always wise to stop using essential oils for an occasional break, and then to continue. I believe this helps stimulate the effect.

Toxicity and Side Effects

Certain citrus oils should not be used just prior to or during sunbathing because they are phototoxic. That means they may produce a change in skin pigmentation on exposure to ultra-violet light. Avoid using bergamot, lemon or lime when sunbathing. Other citrus oils – grapefruit, sweet orange, mandarin/tangerine – have been shown to have only a mild photosensitising effect though it would be as well to be cautious.

All spicy essential oils may irritate sensitive skins but are usually fine if used well-diluted or in a blend.

Large doses of strong relaxing oils, in particular clary sage, can make some people feel drowsy. Do not use such oils on anyone who is soon going to drive a car or use machinery.

Stop using any oil immediately if an adverse reaction is felt.

Patch tests

There is always the chance that a person may be allergic to any essential oil, even though it is one commonly regarded as safe. Anyone susceptible to allergy or who has a sensitive skin should test the oil in weak dilution on a small patch of skin before spreading it over a large area. If there is a skin reaction, do not use it.

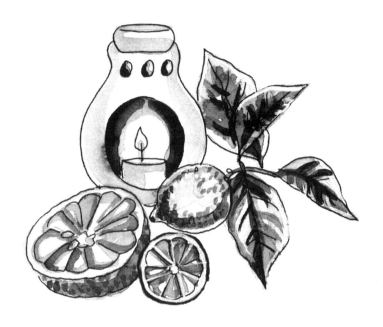

Hazardous oils

Dangerously toxic essential oils are not normally available to the general public, but they are in existence and it is possible that a rogue company might sell them for use in aromatherapy. The list of potentially hazardous essential oils below has been compiled from general information on this subject. Those marked with an asterisk might be used by a professional aromatherapist with specialist knowledge. None of the oils on the list should be used by unqualified people as they could have serious side effects. *This warning applies to the essential oil, and not necessarily to the herb as used in cooking, herbal medicine or homoeopathic remedies.*

Arnica	*Arnica montana*
Bitter almond	*Prunus dulcis var. amara*
Boldo leaf	*Peumus boldus*
Broom	*Cytisus scoparius*
Buchu	*Barosma betulina*
Calamus	*Acorus calamus*
Cinnamon bark	*Cinnamomum cassia*
Camphor, brown and yellow	*Cinnamomum camphora*
*Camphor, white	" "
Chervil	*Anthriscus cerefolium*
Horseradish	*Cochlearia armoracia*
Jaborandi	*Pilocarpus microphyllus*
Melilotus	*Melilotus officinalis*
Mugwort	*Artemisia vulgaris*
Narcissus	*Narcissus poeticus*
Mountain (dwarf) pine	*Pinus mugo (P. pumilio)*
*Pennyroyal	*Mentha pulegium*
Rue	*Ruta graveolens*
Sassafras	*Sassafras variifolium*
Savine	*Juniperus sabina*
Tansy	*Tanacetum vulgare*
Thuja	*Thuja occidentalis*
Tonka	*Diperyx odorata oppositiflora*
Wintergreen	*Gaultheria procumbens*
Wormwood	*Artemisia absinthium*
Wormseed	*Chenopodium ambrosioides*

As the above essential oils are considered hazardous, you may well be asking why they are extracted at all, or listed in books. Many of them are indeed used in perfumes, food flavourings, medicines and medicinal products, but one hopes and assumes that they are harmless in these forms.

There is such a wide choice of essential oils that are safe to use at home that there is no reason to try to find or use any essential oil from the above list.

CHAPTER 6

Methods
of Use

*T*HE quantities of oils specified for the basic preparations in
this chapter are just a guide. If you want to make up less,
simply reduce proportionally the amount of carrier (base) oil
and essential oils given in the formula, and of course use proportionally more if you want to make up a larger quantity. The
quantities given are for adults (see Chapters 10 and 11 for
quantities to use in pregnancy and for children respectively).

Bear in mind that essential oils deteriorate when they are
stored, and you must use suitable bottles to keep them in (see
page 37). If making a small quantity, say about an eggcupful,
you can store it for a couple of days by covering with clingfilm.
For home use, you will probably not need to make up more
than 100 ml of massage oil at a time, which is enough for three
or four whole-body applications.

The amount of base oil needed for a full body massage for a
person of average size is 25 ml, which is roughly equivalent to
two small tablespoons. If you wish to apply a body oil after a
bath or shower you will probably need less than 25 ml, unless
you have a dry skin condition.

A 10 ml dropper bottle is convenient for measuring out
drops of essential oils.

Massage Oils

Quantities: to 50 ml base oil (for example almond *or* 35 ml almond + 15 ml wheatgerm, sesame or vitamin E oils), add approximately 15–20 drops of essential oil. You can use just one essential oil or a combination of up to four.

Example: ten drops of lavender, five drops of sandalwood, five drops of ylang ylang. This is a good combination for a general-purpose oil, for use after a bath or shower. It is relaxing as well as nourishing to the skin. (Use the same quantities if your base is a bland lotion or cream.)

NB: If you wish to use essential oils every day, choose the milder ones and also reduce the recommended amounts by half.

Face Oils

Blend 20 ml at any one time, an amount that should last about one month. Apply face oil three times per week for general skin care, but if you are treating a specific skin complaint use it every night for two or three weeks, then reduce application to three times per week. If you do not like the feel of oil on your face, use a bland lotion or moisturising base.

I find using oil in the mornings very beneficial. This is one of my routines. I wash my face with a very rich honey soap, then I rinse and splash 10–15 times with warm water, pat dry with a towel and immediately apply face oil. By the time I am ready to apply make-up after, say, 20 minutes, the oil has penetrated. I thoroughly blot dry any surface residue and apply a very light matt foundation. Using this method, I have found my make-up looks better and stays on longer.

My favourite face oil is a blend of sandalwood, neroli and lemon. I change the combinations occasionally because the skin gets used to the treatment and needs a boost from time to time.

Essential oils for different skin types

Normal	Cedarwood, geranium, lavender, neroli, patchouli, sandalwood.
Dry	Camomile, clary sage, geranium, jasmine, sandalwood, ylang ylang.
Oily	Bergamot, eucalyptus, juniper, lavender, lemon, lemongrass (in very small doses, test for sensitivity), orange, peppermint, pine, rosemary.
Sensitive	Camomile, jasmine, lavender, rose.
Combination	Cedarwood, clary sage, lavender, ylang ylang.
Mature	Clary sage, frankincense, myrrh, neroli.
Wrinkled	Frankincense, lemon, neroli.

Quantities: To 20 ml base oil (for example almond, or a blend of almond, jojoba and vitamin E), add 10–12 drops of essential oil. For oily skins, try a light coconut oil or grapeseed as the base.

Example: Four drops of lemon, four drops of neroli, four drops of sandalwood (anti-wrinkle formula for mature skins).

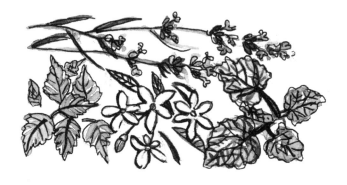

In the Bathroom

Using essential oils in the bath is a pleasurable way of doing oneself good. Essences do not dissolve in water, but that presents no real problem. Just agitate the water vigorously and persistently to disperse the oil. A better way is to take advantage of the oils' solubility in fats. There is fat of course in full-cream milk, and after experimenting with different mediums I decided milk is the best for dissolving essential oils. Add one cup of fresh milk to the water and swish it round. Then add your essential oils, give the water another good swish and imagine you are Cleopatra having your daily bath in asses' milk.

For convenience, you could keep a tin of powdered milk in the bathroom, though not ordinary skimmed milk powder. Full-cream powdered milk is not readily available but there is a skimmed milk on the market containing added vegetable fat which is perfectly suitable (it's what I use). Just half a cup of this in the bath water is sufficient.

For anyone who dislikes the idea of milk in their bath water, an alternative is to put in a tablespoon of a fine-textured vegetable oil, such as almond or grapeseed, and then agitate well. Oil dispersants are also now available.

Do not add essences to hot running water – they will evaporate too quickly. Add them to the water just before you get in, but give it another good swish first.

To gain *maximum* benefit, wash first or take a quick shower. Then add your oils to clean bath water and just soak for 20 minutes in your wonderfully scented milk.

For specific treatments, such as arthritis, stress, depression, skin problems, fatigue and so on, the soaking method is by far the most effective – the introduction of soap to the skin will hinder the absorption of oils. For general use, you can add essences to bubble bath or bath salts.

With a strong sedative oil such as clary sage, it is best to have your bath at a time when you can relax totally afterwards – preferably at night before going to sleep. Four drops should be enough, unless you want to sleep for a week! (It is not advisable to go out immediately after an aromatherapy bath.)

Quantities guide: For adults in normal health, six to eight drops; robust and healthy, up to ten drops; frail adults or of weak constitution, three to four drops. For a baby's bath there are special instructions (see page 139).

After-bath rest periods

Relaxation bath: 1½ hours.

Stimulating bath: 20 minutes – have water cool.

Arthritis/aches and pains/muscular problems: 1 hour.

Depression: 45 minutes–1 hour.

Fatigue, mental or physical: 1–2 hours.

General: 30 minutes.

Aphrodisiac: for two – as long as you like!

Essential oils are extra fast in effect when used in the bath because of absorption through the pores of the skin and by steam inhalation.

Aromatherapy showers

People who have only a shower can make use of one of the following methods or make more use of body oils.

1   Put a flannel over the water outlet and sprinkle about eight drops of essential oil over the shower base. As the steam rises you will inhale the oils.

2   Sprinkle about two or three drops of essence on to a warm, wet flannel and rub briskly over your body (avoiding sensitive areas).

Gargle

To make your own antiseptic gargle, to a cup of warm water add a teaspoonful of honey or salt and one drop of each of the following oils: geranium, lemon, tea-tree, thyme. Stir well to disperse the oils. (If more convenient, use four drops of one.)

Mouthwash

You can make a mouthwash that not only freshens your mouth but is antiseptic and prevents bad breath. See page 175.

Hair conditioner

This is easily made by adding, to a 20 ml bottle of almond, coconut or jojoba oil, ten drops of bay, five drops of lavender and five drops of rosemary. Stand the bottle in a container of hot water for two or three minutes (test the oil for temperature before application). Massage into the hair and scalp, cover your hair with a plastic bag, then a towel, and leave for at least 20 minutes. Finally shampoo thoroughly, rinsing well.

Bidet

For any vaginal or genital irritations, or for haemorrhoids, add four to six drops of essential oils to the water in your bidet or maybe a bowl suitable to sit on. If it is uncomfortable to sit on either for more than five minutes repeat the treatment three or four times a day. It is not necessary to dissolve the essences in milk or almond oil, unless you experience irritation.

Head lice

Mix five drops each of tea-tree and either lavender or geranium into 15ml of almond oil, rub it into the scalp, then comb through before shampooing.

Compresses
~~~~~~~~~~~~~~~

Hot compresses

These are very helpful when an area cannot be treated with oils, lotions or bathing owing to severe inflammation or weeping wounds. They are also very suitable for frail, elderly people. When massage is not advisable, conditions that can be treated with a compress include lumbago (if very painful); slipped disc (should not be massaged); painful, swollen joints; abscesses and boils; earache; period pains; diarrhoea and chest infections (especially in young babies and the elderly).

Large flannels, soft guest towels or lint can be used. The essential oils do not need to be dispersed by agitation of the water as it is necessary for the compress to pick up as much of the essence as possible. The water should be slightly hotter than bath water. Soak the compress, squeezing out excess water. Put the compress on the affected area and keep it in place with perhaps a plastic bag or tinfoil. After the compress has cooled, it should be replaced by a fresh hot one.

Quantities: To two pints hot water add 10–15 drops of oil according to the specific condition. (For sensitive skins, use only six to eight drops; for young children, four drops; babies, one to two drops.)

Cold compresses

Use exactly as in the method above except that the water should be cold from the refrigerator, and the compress can be kept in place with a bandage or plastic bag.

Cold compresses are useful for very inflamed conditions such as swollen arthritic joints, sprains, bruises, stings and bites, inflamed itchy skin, sunburn, headaches, hangovers and jet lag.

Hot and cold compresses

This is an ideal method to relieve sports injuries, especially sprained ankles. If this happens in your household (bloodless injuries), apply neat cajeput or tea-tree. Then as an instant cold compress apply a small packet of frozen peas from your freezer. Shake the peas so that they are loose, mould the packet to the injury and keep in place while you are preparing the hot and cold compresses. Specialist packs of hot or cold compresses are available from clinics, large chemists and health shops.

When the cold compress is prepared, place it over the injury or inflammation. As the compress begins to lose its chill, replace with a hot compress. Do this seven or eight times, ending with a cold compress that can be left in place. If the injury shows no sign of improving, seek medical advice.

If the particular condition is not acute, use compresses over a period of days.

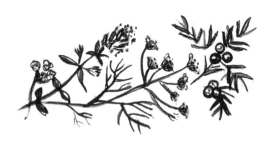

Inhalation

The old-fashioned method, and by far the best, is to use a basin, hot water, essences and a large towel. It is excellent for any breathing difficulties, chest infections, catarrh, sinusitis or headaches.

Pour a pint or two of near-boiling water into a glass or china basin, let the steam subside a little and test it by putting your face over the steam about 25 cm (10in) away. When comfortable, add four or five drops of essential oil to the water and immediately put the towel over your head and the basin, leaving no air holes; keep your eyes closed and breathe in the steam.

You will have to keep coming out for cool air and to blow your nose. If your eyes are sensitive, use sun-bed goggles or eye patches. This method of inhalation can sometimes take your breath away to begin with. Gradually build up inhalation time, starting with 30 seconds' inhalation, then lift the towel, repeat for another 30 seconds, and so on until you have had a total of about five minutes. If possible, inhale for a further full five minutes.

Carefully supervise anyone with a very nervous disposition or who suffers with asthma, and also very young children and the very elderly. If you have broken capillaries (thread veins) on your face, do not use this method too often or for more than two minutes at any one time.

Essence Burners

This is the most versatile and effective method of using essential oils and indeed it is from this that we derive the word 'aromatherapy'. Vaporising is considered by some to be the *only* method and other uses less effective. Inhalation of aromatic vapour certainly introduces the essential oils more quickly into the blood circulation than ingestion and, in some cases, external application. The diffusion of essences is greater and this is therefore considered a safer method of use.

The method of so-called 'burning' essential oils must be carried out correctly. The oils must be in water on a source of heat. As the oil vaporises, its molecules are distributed around us and we inhale the aromatic, moisturised air.

Some essence burners have very shallow dishes suggesting that the essential oil should be dropped, neat, on to the heated pottery or metal. This, in my opinion, is inappropriate for

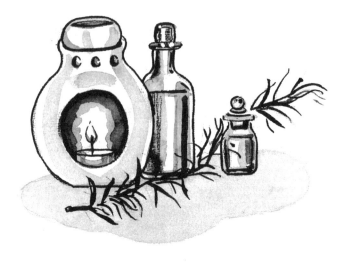

therapy. The overall effect will be aromatic to a degree, but it will be more therapeutic and long-lasting when the essential oils are heated in water. Too much heat denatures the oils.

The source of heat is generally a tiny candle, like a night-light, in a metal container, which is placed in the main body of the burner with enough oxygen circulating to keep the flame at a balanced heat. A word of warning here: night-lights, such as those widely available for use in plate-warmers, fondue sets and vaporisers, are NOT suitable for normal-sized burners as they are too hot; some also have a flashpoint just towards the end of their burning time and are difficult to extinguish. The correct ones for use in most burners are **tea lights**, which are smaller than traditional night-lights, about half the depth, and burn for approximately four hours. Remember not to leave any burner with a lighted candle unattended, especially if you have children or lively pets; if you leave the room, even for a short while, extinguish the candle. The top container should hold just enough water to stay at the right temperature and usually evaporates after approximately two hours. It is advisable not to let the burner run dry (to avoid cracking); top it up with warm water, adding an extra drop or two of oil if necessary.

Some of the really expensive oils (jasmine, neroli, rose) are sold pre-blended with a vegetable oil such as jojoba; these are unsuitable for use in an essence burner.

For specific problems and ailments, blend the recommended oils in a bottle first, then add six to ten drops of the mixture to a little water in the top container. Pre-formulated oils are readily available, saving time and effort.

Use your essence burner for conditions such as depression, tension, anxiety, poor memory, lack of concentration and mental exhaustion. Physical ailments that respond well are headaches, sinusitis, catarrh and respiratory infections (colds, influenza, etc.).

Vaporised essential oils make delightful air fresheners and are completely ozone-friendly. You can create your own personal atmosphere, choosing perhaps clean, fresh, sparkling aromas or even seductive, sexy ones. If you need to put some spice back into your love life, tent the bedroom ceiling with red satin, get some eastern music, dress in a harem costume and blend coriander, sandalwood and ylang ylang in your essence burner. Conversely, if you need to tone down your loving activities, go to bed in curlers, bed socks and enough oil on your face to make you really slippery!

Once you realise the enormous benefits of using an essence burner you will want one in every room. Remember to put it somewhere safe, especially if there are children in the house.

As well as the traditional pottery essence burners, electric burners such as aromastones and aromafans are becoming popular. The principal of vaporising remains the same, but the heat is more constant than relying on candles, and some might think safer. However, they are more expensive, for example some cost over £25, and once the element burns out they are difficult and expensive to repair. Aromastones consist of an electric element contained inside a stone dish, which gets hot and vaporises the essential oils. Although there is no night-light to monitor, you still have to keep an eye on the level of oil, to avoid the nasty smell of oil and water drying out. The aromafans simply pass air over a filter that is impregnated with essential oil, and are therefore more in line with an air freshener than being therapeutic.

Vaporising ring

An alternative means of burning essential oils is the vaporising ring. Although they are widely available from health stores and other outlets, many people do not know how to use them.

Place the ring on a flat surface and put a few drops of perfume oil into the groove. When the ring has absorbed the oil, place it on a light-bulb (60 watt maximum) and switch on the light.

The ring may be used on either a table lamp or on a pendant light (see illustration). In the case of the latter, unscrew the bulb, slip the ring over it and re-screw the bulb into the socket.

This method of vaporising is not as effective as an essence burner for the relief of symptoms, but it's fine if you simply want to create a nice aroma in a room.

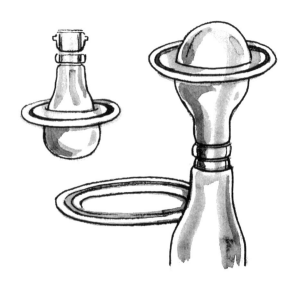

Neat Essential Oils

There are a few instances where essences can be used without preparation.

A few drops of neat lavender oil on your pillow is an effective way to relieve insomnia. Put two or three drops of the oil on either side and in the middle of the pillow, so that when you turn over in the night you'll still get a whiff. Make sure you do not get the oil into your eyes as this will irritate; it should be about 15 cm (6 in) from your nose. Ylang ylang, camomile, marjoram or sandalwood can be used in the same way as lavender. They will not stain (unless adulterated or synthetic).

If you are suffering from a headache or nasal catarrh and you have no access to a burner, put a drop or two of essence on a handkerchief or cotton-wool pad and continually waft it under your nose. Alternatively, put a few drops of essence on your shirt – if it is not an expensive one – about 15 cm (6 in) from your chin.

In an emergency situation, essential oils can be used like smelling salts – pass the bottle just beneath the nose. This procedure can also be used in severe cases of nasal congestion.

Tea-tree oil can be applied neat to athlete's foot and fungal infections of the nails three times a day for about one week until symptoms are relieved.

Dab unsightly pustules, boils and spots with tea-tree or lavender oil on a cotton-wool bud.

Essential oils are a great help in first aid. Some can be used neat for a short time (see page 170).

For Use Around the House

Essential oils can be used either on their own or in conjunction with proprietary household products. Oils of pine, lemon, lavender, orange, tea-tree or thyme can be used as disinfectants.

Add them to hot water for a general wipe-over disinfectant, or to floor-washing/rinsing water. A few drops of lemon, lavender, orange or pine can be dropped into your sink drain or loo.

When washing clothes, essences can be added to the rinsing water (three or four drops to an average-sized bowl) or to your fabric conditioner in the washing machine.

The oils I have mentioned for household use are not expensive, and if you buy large quantities (50 or 100 ml) you will find that most suppliers will give you a discount.

You can easily make your own flower water using essential oils. You will need a large glass bottle (about 200 ml), preferably amber. Use pure spring water and three or four drops of your favourite oil. Choose, for example, from camomile, geranium, jasmine, lavender, lemon, mandarin, neroli, orange (sweet), rose and ylang ylang. Shake the bottle vigorously and keep it in a cool, dark place. Continue to shake it well two or three times a day or every time you pass it. In approximately ten days you will have a lightly perfumed flower water which can be used as a face rinse or spray. Lavender, camomile, rose, lemon or orange water can be used in the making of sweets such as fondants or icings.

For Animals

To bathe a wound or abscess, to half a pint of cooled boiled water add three drops of lavender, or four drops of tea-tree, or three drops of lemon oil, or a dessertspoon of pure freshly squeezed (not bottled) lemon juice.

To get rid of fleas, tea-tree or garlic oil should be rubbed on your hands and then rubbed through the fur of your dog or cat (they don't like the smell too much, but neither do the fleas!). The oils are non-poisonous and will not hurt the animal when it grooms itself but garlic may make it difficult for the cat to find a welcoming lap.

Oil of citronella sprinkled around your garden plants is reputed to stop pussy digging. Hiding strips of paper impregnated with citronella may stop determined claws being exercised on your carpets or chairs (you will have to impregnate the strips regularly as the aroma wears off). You can buy scratching posts for your beloved moggy impregnated with cat mint: the cat obligingly sharpens its claws on the post and not on your furniture. But my ginger Tom slobbers, cuddles, sits and sleeps on his catmint post and wouldn't dream of scratching it – only armchairs are good enough for that.

A drop of neat lavender or tea-tree can be administered as first aid directly on to a scratch or shallow cut. To relieve arthritis or rheumatism gently massage your pet with a few drops of an essential oil, or a combination of oils, added to white lotion, grapeseed oil, or light coconut oil. Oils such as cajeput, marjoram, eucalyptus, camomile, lavender, black pepper, ginger and tea-tree will help stiff and painful legs and joints. If there is fluid present or a great deal of inflammation, try compresses of cajeput and lemon.

For skin problems such as eczema, try tea-tree and juniper in compresses, or in a base of white lotion or cream.

For cystitis, try a combination of two drops of tea-tree, two drops of eucalyptus, two drops of sandalwood in a teaspoon of lotion or oil. Rub this around the cat's or dog's outlet. They promptly lick it off, but this gets the oils into the system and helps to cure the problem. Do this twice a day until symptoms are relieved.

Animals suffering from anxiety following a trauma will benefit from the use of soothing oils such as camomile and bergamot in a burner (placed safely out of reach).

Do not use aromatherapy if the animal urgently needs veterinary treatment, or if symptoms persist or if the animal shows signs of distress.

71

Getting to Know Essential Oils

*B*ECAUSE there are so many essential oils on the market, it is difficult to know where to start and end. This chapter deals, in some detail, with 44 of the more popular and well-known essential oils, which have also proved to be invaluable in my aromatherapy practice. In my opinion, they are all suitable for home use, provided all instructions are followed. They present a varied and useful selection and are widely available. However, if you have difficulty in obtaining any of them, details of some reputable suppliers are given on pages 218–9.

Before using any essential oils, it is very important to read the cautions given in Chapter 5 and also those listed against individual oils. This will prevent unnecessary problems, such as skin irritation or minor side effects.

Active Principles and Properties

BASIL *(Ocimum basilicum)*
The oil is extracted from the leaves and flowers of a very familiar herb. The essential oil contains methyl chavicol, which has caused some controversy over its use. The French (or Egyptian) oil is the best to use and it has such beneficial effects I believe that it is invaluable, provided all necessary cautions are

observed. It has a wonderful sweet herbaceous aroma, and reminds me of fresh pea pods.

Methods of use: bath (low dosage), essence burner, massage oil (low dosage).

Caution: use in moderation. Might irritate sensitive skin. Avoid during pregnancy.

Action: antidepressant, antiseptic, antispasmodic, cephalic (head-related), digestive, emmenagogue, expectorant, restorative, tonic.

Healing effects: basil has been used for thousands of years especially in ayurvedic (traditional Hindu) medicine. It is used as an antidote to poisonous snake or insect bites, as well as traditionally being used as a remedy for colds and flu. It is also very effective for problems affecting breathing, such as asthma, bronchitis, emphysema and shallow breathing due to stress. Basil is used to help depression and insomnia caused by stress and anxiety, can ease aches and pains in muscles and joints and is effective in cases of gout. It is at its most effective when used to treat the mind, where it is strengthening and brings clarity to thoughts. It is effective to treat depression and confusion, as well as feelings of resentment. It is uplifting and is a tonic to the nervous system.

BENZOIN *(Styrax benzoin)*
Benzoin is a gum resin extracted from a large tropical tree. The tree exudes the gum from cuts in the bark and the resinoid is extracted by solvent. Benzoin is used in pharmaceutical products, perfumes and cosmetics. It has an aroma reminiscent of vanilla.

Methods of use: essence burner, inhalation, massage oil.

Caution: do not use on very sensitive or damaged skin. Avoid during early pregnancy.

Action: anti-inflammatory, antiseptic, antifungal, expectorant, sedative.

Healing effects: benzoin has been used for thousands of years as an incense and as a medicine. It is traditionally used for its effect on the respiratory tract as an antiseptic and expectorant. Benzoin is helpful to most conditions affecting the lungs, bronchial tubes, throat and sinuses and is soothing to painful joints caused by arthritis, rheumatism and poor circulation. It is effective in relieving stress, anxiety and depression by creating a relaxing and protective energy in times of distress. It calms the mind and helps meditation.

BERGAMOT *(Citrus bergamia)*
An olive-green oil obtained by expression or steam distillation from the peel of a citrus fruit native to Calabria in southern Italy. The plant is a small tree and should not be confused with the herbaceous plant of the same name, which is also called bee balm (*Monarda* species). Its lively fresh aroma is quite distinctive – it is the scent in Earl Grey tea, and is also used in eau de Cologne.

Methods of use: bath, essence burner, massage oil (test skin for sensitivity).

Caution: this oil is phototoxic, so do not use it whilst sunbathing or before exposing yourself to the sun. Do not use the oil if there are raised moles on the skin. Bergamot can irritate sensitive skins. For regular skin application, use Bergamot FCF (fourocoumarin free) – it is safer for use on skin. Expressed Bergamot is not recommended. Distilled is a lighter green.

Action: antispasmodic, antidepressant, deodorant, expectorant, nerve tonic.

Healing effects: uplifting, calming and relaxing without a sedative effect. Gives a sensation of slow motion, rather like floating. Promotes a feeling of love and peace. I find it helps with problems of indecision, as well as bringing harmony and balance to the psyche (inner mind/soul). It relieves tension, anxiety, extreme negativity and depression. Use it especially when there is a need to release emotional stress. It is thought that bergamot regulates thyroid gland activity.

In massage oils or lotions, bergamot can heal skin problems, such as eczema, psoriasis, acne and oily conditions. For this purpose it is best mixed with other oils (see recipe sections in Chapter 13).

For sore throats and bad breath, bergamot can be used in a gargle or mouthwash (do not swallow).

Treat bronchitis with chest rubs or inhalation.

BLACK PEPPER *(Piper nigrum)*

The essential oil is extracted from the berries of a woody vine. The berries start off red and turn black as they mature, and are known as peppercorns. The aroma is warm and spicy.

Methods of use: bath (very low dosage, one or two drops), essence burner, massage oil or lotion.

Caution: will irritate sensitive skin, so use in low dosage and moderate frequency. Avoid use if conditions such as diverticulitis, ulcerative colitis, or any inflammatory bowel condition exist. Avoid during the first six months of pregnancy.

Action: analgesic, antiseptic, antispasmodic, expectorant, rubifacient.

Healing effects: due to the rubifacient effect, black pepper is warming and stimulating to the circulation, thus easing aches and pains and muscular tension caused by arthritis, rheumatism, sports activity and gardening. Whilst black pepper can have a stimulating effect on the bowels, it also calms diarrhoea caused by bacteria.

Because of its stimulating effect, it is wise not to use black pepper directly on the abdomen in cases of inflammation, but it can be used on joints or localised sites of muscular pain. Black pepper is helpful in cases of mental fatigue and will also assist in cases of emotional exhaustion. Blended with lemongrass, it will clear a negative and heavy atmosphere.

CAJEPUT *(Melaleuca leucadendron, M. minor)*
This colourless or very pale yellow oil comes from the leaves and twigs of a medium-sized tree native to India. It has a powerful, fresh, herbaceous scent with eucalyptus tones.

Methods of use: bath, compress, essence burner, massage oil.

Caution: can cause slight irritation to sensitive skins. Avoid use in early pregnancy.

Action: analgesic, antiseptic, rubefacient, stimulant.

Healing effects: cajeput is one of the best natural analgesics. It blends and works well with other oils and can also be used successfully on its own. For toothache, add five or six drops of cajeput to a warm compress and apply to the face around the affected area. This will dull the pain. For sprains and bruises, apply a little neat oil as first aid only. In the long term, treat with diluted oil either in compresses or lotions.

The oil has a mild diuretic effect on injuries that are prone to fluid build-up.

Other physical conditions that may respond well to cajeput include: acne, arthritis, asthma, bronchitis, dental neuralgia, dermatitis, earache, eczema, gout, headaches, laryngitis, period pains, psoriasis, rheumatism, sore throats and torn ligaments. Use cajeput diluted in almond oil to soothe sunburn.

Mentally, cajeput has a stimulating, invigorating effect. I find this oil works well on emotions when dealing with a painful experience, whether recent or long past.

CAMOMILE, TRUE (ROMAN) *(Chamaemelum nobile,* formerly *Anthemis nobilis)*
and
CAMOMILE, WILD (GERMAN) *(Matricaria recutita,* formerly *M. chamomilla, Chamomilla recutita)*

These two species of camomile are widely used in aromatherapy and their properties are very similar. The oil is extracted by steam distillation from the flowers of German camomile and from the whole plant of Roman camomile. The oil of the former species is deep blue and the aroma is sweet herbaceous, like strong honey, with fruity undertones. The oil of the latter is paler and a greener blue, the aroma being sweet herbaceous, and like tea. The blue colour of camomile oil turns green with age. German camomile contains chamazulene, which makes it very effective for skin problems, ulcers, infected or inflamed conditions such as cellulitis (inflammation of cells).

Methods of use: bath, compress, essence burner, massage oil or lotion.

Caution: a mild emmenagogue; avoid during early pregnancy.

Action: antiseptic, analgesic, anti-inflammatory, antispasmodic, astringent, diuretic, emmenagogue, febrifuge, hepatic, sedative.

Healing effects: the healing effect of camomile on the skin is due to a blue substance called azulene that it contains (especially the German camomile). It eases inflammation, eruptions or ulceration such as acne, burns, eczema and psoriasis.

The herb was used in folk medicine to reduce fevers. In aromatherapy it is effective in treating the following physical conditions: arthritis and rheumatism, digestive problems, liver congestion, muscular cramps and spasm. It may also be used for period irregularities, pre-menstrual tension (PMT) and menopausal problems.

It has a soothing and calming effect both on irritable children and grumpy adults. Anger, rage, anguish, severe tension and obsessiveness are negative emotions that may be alleviated by this oil. Roman camomile is very effective for emotional healing

CEDARWOOD, ATLAS *(Cedrus atlantica)*
and
CEDARWOOD, RED (VIRGINIAN) *(Juniper virginiana)*

The oil of more than one type of tree is sold as cedarwood. The Atlas cedar is a true cedar and closely related to the cedar of Lebanon (*Cedrus libani*), which unfortunately no longer grows in abundance (only a few hundred survive). The oil from the wood is pale yellow. It has a soft, warm woody fragrance, with sandalwood undertones that are sweeter and stronger. Red (Virginian) cedarwood oil is recognised by its very woody aroma reminiscent of pencils.

Method of use: bath, essence burner, massage oil or lotion.

Caution: Virginian cedarwood oil is abortive and should not be used during pregnancy. Atlas cedar is an immuno-stimulant (see cautionary notes on page 50).

Action: antiseptic, astringent, diuretic, expectorant, sedative.

Healing effects: oil of cedarwood, as an astringent, is good for acne and oily skin conditions, eczema and psoriasis. Mixed with lemon oil, it helps relieve sinusitis and breathing difficulties such as catarrh and bronchitis. It is a remedy for urinary infections, helps stress-related conditions and is also useful as a stimulant in cases of low sexual response due to nervous tension.

Cedarwood uplifts the spirit and aids meditation. The mental effect is sedative, harmonising, strengthening and soothing. If you suffer from low self-esteem or lack confidence, cedarwood may help. It is also helpful in cases of arthritis and rheumatism.

CITRONELLA *(Cymbopogen nardus)*

This oil is extracted from an aromatic grass which mainly comes from Ceylon and Java. It has a sweet lemony fragrance, and is widely used in perfumed products, air fresheners and disinfectants.

Methods of use: essence burner, massage oil (very low dosage).

Caution: can cause skin irritation, avoid direct contact. Avoid during pregnancy.

Action: antidepressant, anti-inflammatory, antiseptic, deodorant, emmenagogue, insecticide.

Healing effects: citronella has an uplifting effect and is helpful in cases of mild depression. It can also be effective in relieving fatigue, headaches, migraine, head colds and flu, as well as minor infections. It is widely used as a repellent against mosquitoes and other flying intruders. It has also been discovered that cats do not like the aroma of citronella, and is sold in garden centres to deter unwanted moggies from digging up your favourite plants. Used in a burner, it clears unpleasant smells around the house.

CLARY SAGE *(Salvia sclarea)*

The plant is in the same family as the common sage (*Salvia officinalis*), the oil of which is considered toxic and is not recommended for general use. Clary sage, however, is comparatively free from toxicity. Obtained from the flowering tops, it is pale yellow with a herbaceous, hay-like aroma, warm, musky and strong.

Methods of use: bath, essence burner, massage oil or lotion.

Caution: use in moderation. Large amounts can cause drowsiness. Avoid during pregnancy, if on oestrogen supplements or if suffering with uterine or ovarian growths or cancer.

Action: antidepressant, antiseptic, antispasmodic, astringent, emmenagogue, sedative, stimulates hormones.

Healing effects: clary sage is renowned for its sedative effect. The drowsiness it might cause can last for several days. However, after it has had time to reduce anxiety, it becomes restorative to the whole system, recharging the emotional and physical batteries. Use less clary sage than other oils because it is very strong.

A clary sage bath before going to bed will help dissolve any stress and muscular tension. I find clary sage benefits mature skins.

Clary sage is helpful with PMT and menopausal problems. To ease period pains, mix clary sage with cajeput and camomile in a massage oil or lotion and apply to the abdomen. Alternatively, use the same essential oils in a warm compress. During labour, use a clary sage compress on the abdomen, and a few drops in the burner.

For troubled sleep, massage the solar plexus area (middle diaphragm, just below the ribs) and the feet with diluted clary sage and lavender.

Clary sage is wonderful at times of extreme anguish, depression, panic or shock; it will help to put problems in perspective. Use it for mental and physical debility.

CORIANDER *(Coriandrum sativum)*

The oil is extracted mainly from the crushed ripe seeds of the herb. Extractions may be made from the whole plant, sometimes referred to as Chinese parsley. The aroma is warm and spicy.

Methods of use: bath, essence burner, massage oil or lotion.

Caution: may irritate sensitive skin. Avoid use if on oestrogen supplements. Avoid during pregnancy. Avoid if on HRT.

Action: analgesic, anti-inflammatory, antirheumatic, antispasmodic, digestive, hormonal.

Healing effects: like all spices, coriander is warming and stimulating and relieves any problems of the digestive tract; a few drops in a base oil rubbed gently into the abdomen eases discomfort due to bacteria, wind or constipation. It is also helpful and effective in reducing aches and pains due to the accumulation of toxins caused by arthritis and rheumatism. It has a stimulating effect on the hormones and is therefore effective in cases of irregular periods, PMT and menopause.

Coriander is also helpful in cases of nervous exhaustion and mental fatigue and can work very well to relieve stress. One of my favourite soups is carrot and coriander, and I find the colour and flavour totally therapeutic and uplifting, as well as delicious. Use the whole herb rather than the oil in cooking as the flavour is more delicate.

CYPRESS, ITALIAN *(Cupressus sempervirens)*
This cypress is native to the Mediterranean region. The pale yellow, almost colourless oil is distilled from the needles, twigs and cones. Its refreshing aroma, similar to pine, is a little spicy with woody tones.

Methods of use: bath, bidet, essence burner, footbath, massage oil or lotion.

Caution: avoid during pregnancy; avoid if uterine or ovarian growths or cancer are present.

Action: antiseptic, antispasmodic, astringent, deodorant, diuretic, nerve tonic, stimulates hormones.

Healing effects: cypress has been used in medicine for thousands of years and was thought to be a remedy used by Hippocrates (the father of medicine). The oil has a warming, balancing effect on the body systems and is relaxing without causing drowsiness. It has a refreshing, uplifting and regenerating effect, calming irritability and impatience. Cypress can sometimes help with indecision.

The oil has an astringent effect on haemorrhoids and varicose veins. It alleviates menstrual and menopausal problems. For hot flushes, before going to bed, try a foot massage with equal parts of cypress and clary sage diluted in almond oil.

Use cypress as a skin tonic for an oily skin, and in a footbath when there is an odour problem.

DILL *(Anethum graveolens)*

The oil is extracted from the seeds and weed of the whole plant, and has been traditionally used for thousands of years as a culinary herb in fish dishes, bread and pickles.

Methods of use: bath, essence burner, massage oil or lotion.

Caution: may irritate highly sensitive skins. Avoid during pregnancy.

Action: antiseptic, antispasmodic, digestive, diuretic, emmenagogue.

Healing effects: whilst dill is not widely used in aromatherapy treatment, it is a helpful oil to have on hand to relieve cases of stomach upsets, colic, dyspepsia and indigestion. It is also helpful in cases of fluid retention, and effective in cases of scanty or missing periods. Dill also helps promote the flow of milk in nursing mothers. The essential oil should not be taken internally due to the concentration factor, but the plant is used in pharmaceutical preparations such as 'dill water' or 'gripe water'.

EUCALYPTUS *(Eucalyptus globulus)*

The hundreds of species of eucalyptus are mostly native to Australia. They range in height from small shrubs under ten feet to the tallest known broad-leafed tree (*E. regnans*) reaching nearly 400 feet. The oil most frequently used in aromatherapy comes from *E. globulus*, otherwise known as the southern blue gum, which can grow to over 100 feet tall. Almost colourless, this oil, which comes from the leaves and twigs, has a very powerful, readily recognisable smell with a camphoraceous note.

Methods of use: bath, essence burner, inhalant, massage oil.

Cautions: avoid if epileptic or suffering from high blood pressure; avoid in early pregnancy.

Action: analgesic, antiseptic, antispasmodic, deodorant, diuretic, expectorant, mental stimulant, rubefacient.

Healing effects: eucalyptus is an age-old remedy for colds and flu, due to its decongestant, anti-viral and bactericidal action. It is also helpful in urinary tract infections, asthma, rheumatism and for muscular aches and pains and is an effective insect repellant.

The psychological effect of eucalyptus can be described as stimulating and uplifting. If you are feeling lethargic or low in spirits, eucalyptus may be just what you need.

FENNEL, SWEET *(Foeniculum vulgare)*

The oil from this herb, native to the Mediterranean region, is extracted from the seeds by steam distillation. Very pale yellow in colour, it has a sweet aroma that is delicate but penetrating, and reminiscent of aniseed.

Methods of use: bath, essence burner, massage oil.

Caution: use in moderation. Large doses over a long period could produce side effects. The oil should not be used on very young children or on sensitive skin. It should not be used by people with epilepsy. Avoid during pregnancy and if on oestrogen supplements. Avoid if uterine or ovarian growths or cancer are present.

Action: antiseptic, antispasmodic, carminative, emmenagogue, expectorant, digestive, diuretic, stimulant.

Healing effects: fennel has been used in medicine for thousands of years and was believed to impart strength and fortitude. Eating the seed helped dispel flatulence. It was also supposed to reduce obesity and promote the flow of milk in nursing mothers. Its hormonal effect is used to relieve menopausal and menstrual problems. Use a few drops of fennel in almond oil as a soothing massage oil for the abdomen.

Fennel oil used either in the bath or as a massage rub reduces excess fluid caused by hormonal imbalances (fennel tea should be drunk as well). It is valuable in the treatment of cellulite.

Fennel may be used in cases of weakness of character, insecurity, fear, worry and moodiness.

FRANKINCENSE *(Boswellia carterii)*
Also known as olibanum, or sometimes gum thus, it is extracted by steam distillation from the resin of a small African tree. The oil is amber or greeny-yellow in colour with a warm, spicy, slightly peppery scent.

Methods of use: bath, compress, essence burner, lotion or massage oil.

Cautions: avoid during pregnancy.

Action: antiseptic, astringent, cicatrising, diuretic, sedative, tonic.

Healing effects: frankincense is exceptional for skin care, revitalising and rejuvenating the tissues, giving a healthy glow and keeping wrinkles at bay. For excessive menstrual bleeding, I recommend using frankincense in a compress, or diluted in an almond oil base and gently applied to the abdomen.

Thousands of years ago, frankincense was used in rituals for purification and the exorcism of evil spirits. I believe that frankincense has the same effect on our bodies and minds, cleansing negative thoughts – fear, resentment, worry and confusion – and replacing them with a feeling of well-being and tranquillity.

GERANIUM *(Pelargonium odorantissimum, P. graveolens, P. capitatum* and other species)*

This essential oil is derived from the geraniums grown in garden tubs and window-boxes, more correctly named pelargoniums, and very widely cultivated. Obtained by steam distillation, the oil is a pale soft green with a sweet floral scent that varies depending on the species used.

Methods of use: bath, essence burner, massage oil or lotion.

Caution: may irritate very sensitive skins. Avoid in early pregnancy.

Action: antidepressant, antiseptic, astringent, circulatory stimulant, diuretic, hypotensive, sedative, tonic.

Healing effects: geranium oil stimulates the adrenal glands, promoting natural balance of the hormones, which is a great help for menopause troubles and pre-menstrual tension.

The oil is particularly useful in many types of skin conditions: burns, ulcers, wounds, dermatitis, eczema, psoriasis and inflammation.

The effect of geranium oil on the mind is calming and uplifting. It strengthens the personality by increasing confidence and self-esteem. The oil combats mood swings, tension, tearfulness and depression.

GINGER *(Zinziber officinale)*
The oil is extracted from the rhizomes (roots) of the plant, which is a perennial herb. Ginger root is traditionally used as a culinary spice and is sometimes crystallised and served as a sweet. It has the most delicious sweet and spicy aroma.

Methods of use: bath, essence burner, massage oil or lotion.

Caution: may irritate sensitive skin. Avoid in early pregnancy.

Action: analgesic, antiseptic, antispasmodic, digestive, expectorant, rubefacient, stimulant.

Healing effects: stimulating and warming to the system, ginger is an invaluable oil to have around the house. It is antiseptic and helps relieve the symptoms of colds and flu and minor infections. It is very effective for the relief of muscular aches and pains, and stiffness in the joints caused by arthritis, rheumatism and the menopause. Whilst ginger is a mild laxative, I have found it invaluable in cases of diarrhoea. Mix six to eight drops of ginger in two teaspoons of base oil and gently massage into the abdomen, repeating every few hours until symptoms have eased. This works in cases of mild food poisoning and stress reaction. If symptoms persist, or are accompanied by sweating and vomiting, seek immediate medical treatment. Ginger is very effective in cases of mental fatigue and mild depression; it imparts strength and warmth and encourages positive energy.

GRAPEFRUIT *(Citrus paradisi)*
Essential oil of grapefruit, obtained from the peel, is becoming increasingly popular among aromatherapists. It comes mainly from the USA and has a fresh, bright, tangy aroma just like the fruit.

Methods of use: bath, essence burner, massage oil or lotion.

Caution: can irritate sensitive skins and is mildly phototoxic. Do not use on raised skin moles.

Action: diuretic, general stimulant, lymphatic stimulant, tonic.

Healing effects: grapefruit uplifts mind, body and spirit. It combats both physical and mental tiredness – jet lag in particular – restoring energy levels. It feels very cooling in hot weather. You will find it helpful in common ailments such as fluid retention due to overweight, pre-menstrual tension and menopausal problems. It also stimulates the lymphatic system and helps eliminate toxins. Use it to ease anxiety and lift depression; it can clear confusion and indecision, and sharpens the mind.

The oil is also useful for freshening rooms, especially after smokers have been in them. It reduces animal odours and cooking smells.

JASMINE *(Jasminum officinale, J. grandiflorum)*
Jasmine absolute is extremely expensive. Large quantities of flowers are needed to produce a small amount of oil. However, its exquisite aroma – sweet, floral, with almost harsh honey-like tones – is so strong that very little is needed. It is dark brown in colour.

Methods of use: bath, face oil, lotion. If you feel extravagant, it can be used in an essence burner. However, the oil is mostly sold in a jojoba base which is not suitable for burning.

Caution: avoid in early pregnancy.

Action: antidepressant, antiseptic, antispasmodic, sedative.

Healing effects: like rose oil, jasmine has a wonderful effect on the skin, regardless of type or age. Jasmine relaxes muscles that are stiff and tight from anxiety and tension and is wonderfully relaxing when used in the bath. Often people who suffer from extreme anguish are so-called chilly mortals; this chilliness is caused by blocked energy. Jasmine is of great help in warming the spirit and releasing any such blockages. Regular use of jasmine helps raise self-esteem, increases confidence and imparts a feeling of well-being.

Jasmine is believed to stimulate creativity and original ideas! Used at night, it induces sleep and brings forth wonderful dreams.

JUNIPER BERRY *(Juniperus communis)*

Juniper is an evergreen shrub-like plant, and the oil is extracted from the ripe black berries. It has been used for centuries in medicine to treat respiratory and urinary tract conditions. The aroma is very reminiscent of gin.

Methods of use: bath, essence burner, massage oil or lotion.

Caution: use in moderation. Avoid use if suffering from debilitating kidney or bladder disease. Avoid totally during pregnancy. May irritate sensitive skin.

Action: antirheumatic, antiseptic, antispasmodic, antitoxin, diuretic, emmenagogue, rubifacient, sedative.

Healing effects: juniper is helpful to conditions caused by the accumulation of toxins and uric acid, for example cellulite and sluggish lymphatic circulation, arthritis and gout. It also reduces fluid retention by its diuretic action. Whilst it is very effective against mild infections of the urinary tract such as cystitis, it should be avoided by sufferers of kidney disease due to the stimulating and nephrotoxic effects. Juniper is also very helpful to skin conditions such as eczema, psoriasis and acne. It is also widely used in aromatherapy for its sedative action and is effective in treating stress and anxiety. It restores energy and is generally uplifting.

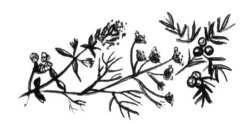

LAVANDIN *(Lavandula* hybrid*)*

The essential oil is extracted from the leaves, flowers and twigs of the whole plant. Lavandin has been developed by crossing lavender (*L. angustifolia*) and spike lavender (*L. latifolia*). The aroma is very like lavender, but with a slightly more camphoraceous note. It is widely used in toiletries and soaps.

Methods of use: bath, essence burner, massage oil or lotion.

Caution: avoid during early pregnancy.

Action: antidepressant, anti-inflammatory, antiseptic, expectorant, mild emmenagogue, tonic.

Healing effects: there are great similarities in the action and effect of lavandin and lavender, and the two are easily interchangeable. However, lavandin is more effective for the treatment of muscular aches, pains and cramp and conditions affecting the respiratory system. Lavandin is also stimulating to the blood circulation and helps to eliminate toxins. It is not so sedative as lavender and can be more helpful for stress in the work-place. It has a calming soothing effect, but does not induce sleepiness. It is refreshing to a tired mind and imparts peaceful thoughts.

LAVENDER *(Lavandula angustifolia,* also known as *L. officinalis* and *L. spica).*

The common or old English lavender originated in the Mediterranean region but is grown commercially in several countries, including England and France. Its delightful aroma is familiar to everyone. The oil, colourless or pale yellow, is obtained by steam distillation and could be described as herbaceous and floral with woody undertones.

See also Lavandin.

Methods of use: bath, compresses, essence burner, lotion, massage oil. It can also be used neat as first aid. A drop or two on the pillow will aid restful sleep.

Caution: a mild emmenagogue; avoid in early pregnancy.

Action: analgesic, antiseptic, antispasmodic, cicatrising, deodorant, diuretic, emmenagogue, expectorant, hypotensive, sedative.

Healing effects: a favourite aromatic for thousands of years, there certainly do not appear to be many conditions lavender cannot help. Versatile and safe, it is ideal for home use. Keep a bottle handy for all kinds of emergencies. In the event of a cut, burn, bite or sting, apply neat lavender oil directly on the affected part – it will rapidly relieve pain and heal the tissue. Lavender will act as a bactericidal agent for the treatment of acne. Apply neat oil to the spot with the tip of a cotton-wool bud. Although safe to use neat on a troubled area, lavender will dry the skin if over-used.

After many years of using it, I am still amazed at how many everyday problems good old lavender helps. It can soothe and calm all kinds of nervous tension and shock, helping to lift depression, dispel irritability, and quell panic and hysteria. A few drops rubbed on the forehead soothes a headache. Try it to alleviate muscular aches and pains, arthritic and rheumatic pain, cramp, dermatitis, eczema, dry skin, oily skin, sunburn, sinusitis, colds, influenza, bronchitis, asthma, high blood pressure, insomnia, mental debility and anxiety.

LEMON *(Citrus limonum)*

The lemon tree, a native of south-east Asia, was introduced to Italy about some 1,500 years ago, whence its cultivation has spread throughout the Mediterranean region and to other parts of the world. The greenish-yellow oil is expressed from the rind.

Methods of use: bath, essence burner, massage oil or lotion. The juice of a lemon can be used neat as an antiseptic, or diluted in water as a gargle.

Caution: citrus oils can cause skin irritations and are photo-toxic (see page 54).

Action: antiseptic, astringent, diuretic (mild), expectorant, hepatic, hypotensive, mental stimulant, tonic.

Healing effects: lemon is a very important essential oil and, like lavender, it helps numerous conditions. Because of its antiseptic action, lemon oil is useful for treating respiratory tract infections – colds, sore throats, influenza, bronchitis and sinusitis. For tonsillitis, gargle with lemon juice in warm water. Bathe infected wounds with diluted lemon juice or oil. It can relieve heaches and migraine (try slices of lemon on the forehead).

Lemon stimulates the circulation and is therefore considered helpful in treating varicose veins.

Traditionally, lemon juice is squeezed over fish and shellfish, as it combats bacterial contamination. We are constantly being warned about the dangers of pathogenic bacteria in the foods that we buy, so I always cook poultry and fish with whole lemons, plenty of garlic and fresh rosemary.

Try oil of lemon to ease asthma, gingevitis (inflammation of the gums) and liverishness, and to help get rid of warts, verrucas, and vaginal thrush.

For skin care, essential oil of lemon added to almond oil or a bland cream acts as a cleanser, toner and a great anti-wrinkle agent. A drop of the oil added to toothpaste will keep your teeth sparkling white.

Lemon oil has a stabilising effect on the emotions and helps treat anxiety. Inhaling the vapour of lemon oil connects the spirit and the body to the higher self.

LEMONGRASS *(Cymbopogen citratus)*

The essential oil is extracted from a fragrant and aromatic tropical grass, mainly from India and Guatemala. The grass is widely used in cooking and is now a familiar sight in supermarkets. The aroma of lemongrass from Cochin differs slightly from the grass from Guatamala. Cochin lemongrass is strong and lemony but with a herbaceous tone, whereas the grass from Guatamala has a distinctively sweet, sharp, lemony aroma. Lemongrass is often mistaken for lemon verbena (*Lippia citriodora*) which in fact is a herb.

Methods of use: essence burner.

Caution: lemongrass is a skin irritant, and so not always tolerated in a bath or oil. Try a patch test first. Avoid in early pregnancy.

Action: antidepressant, antiseptic, astringent, antidepressant, deodorant, fungicide, insect repellent, tonic (nervous system).

Healing effects: because of its effects on certain skin types, lemongrass is sometimes avoided as a massage oil or bath treatment, but if your skin will accept the oil it has a marvellous restorative and uplifting effect. It is also very good for the treatment of sports injuries and torn ligaments. It has a toning and stimulating effect on muscles and can help reduce the effects of oily skin conditions. Used in a burner, lemongrass can ease tension headaches. If you suffer from headaches caused by perfumes or aromas in general, use lemongrass in moderation. It is most effective when used to promote psychic studies, development, and psychic protection. It imparts a feeling of freshness and well-being.

MANDARIN (*Citrus reticulata*)
The oil is extracted by steam distillation of the pulped fruit, and smells exactly like the fruit.

Methods of use: bath, essence burner, massage oil or lotion.

Caution: mildly phototoxic, avoid when sunbathing.

Action: antiseptic, antispasmodic, diuretic (mild), laxative (mild), sedative.

Healing effects: mandarin has a delicious aroma and is immediately calming and uplifting. It has a strong antiseptic effect and is very acceptable to children as it is an aroma they know and trust. Good for tummy upsets, especially caused by anxiety, it has a mild laxative effect and will help young constipated tummies. Mandarin is helpful when on a diet as it encourages the appetite for citrus fruits and gently reduces fluid retention. It is an oil that can be safely used during pregnancy and will aid restful sleep. It calms anxiety and restlessness, uplifting the spirit.

MARJORAM, SWEET *(Origanum marjorana)*
A pale yellowish, spicy oil is obtained from the flowering tops and leaves of this well-known European herb.

Methods of use: bath, essence burner, massage oil or lotion, drops on pillow.

Caution: over-use could cause a stupefying effect. Avoid during pregnancy. Avoid if being treated for clinical depression (see page 51).

Action: analgesic, antiseptic, antispasmodic, emmenagogue, expectorant, sedative.

Healing effects: marjoram has a warming effect on the body which is effective on muscular spasm, arthritis and rheumatism. Mix it with lavender, camomile and cajeput, to make a soothing lotion to relieve the pain of all kinds of muscular problems, especially cramp.

The oil often alleviates headaches and migraine, and calms the digestive system.

Marjoram has a soothing and fortifying effect on the mind and in times of grief can impart warmth and strength. It will also help feelings of loneliness and sorrow (but see caution above).

MELISSA (LEMON BALM) *(Melissa officinalis)*
Native to southern Europe, though widely grown elsewhere, the lemon balm plant yields only minute quantities of oil. This makes it difficult to obtain and also extremely expensive to buy. World production can be as little as two kilograms. However, it is possible to purchase a therapeutically identical melissa oil reconstructed out of the natural plant components. This is considered to be a reconstructed oil, not a synthetic. It has a sharp, sweet, strong lemon aroma.

Sometimes melissa is cut with lemongrass or citronella. A synthetically produced melissa oil is supplied to the perfume industry – one hopes this type is never sold to aromatherapists. Lemon or lemongrass is often mixed with the genuine oil to bring down the cost.

Methods of use: bath, essence burner, massage oil or lotion.

Caution: can irritate very sensitive skins. Avoid during early pregnancy.

Action: antispasmodic, digestive, sedative, tonic.

Healing effects: uplifting, calming, soothing, the herb has been used for hundreds of years as an 'elixir of life'. A heart tonic, melissa also relieves symptoms of anxiety, panic and shock. It clears the mind and raises the spirits.

You can enjoy melissa as a herbal tea. Steep one ounce (25 grams) of the leaves in one pint of boiling water. Let the tea stand for 15–20 minutes. Add honey and drink either warm or chilled.

Melissa may be considered safe to use throughout pregnancy.

MYRRH *(Commiphora myrrha)*
Myrrh is an oleo gum resin and the oil is extracted from the dried gum which exudes from the cut bark. The shrub grows mainly in north-east Africa, and has been used for thousands of years as both medicine and perfume. It was a substance prized

by the queens of ancient Egypt for its magical properties for incense and beauty care.

Methods of use: bath, essence burner, massage oil or cream, tincture.

Caution: avoid use during pregnancy.

Action: anticatarrhal, anti-inflammatory, antiseptic, astringent, emmenagogue, expectorant, fungicide, sedative, skin tonic.

Healing effects: myrrh has traditionally been used in medicines that help conditions affecting the respiratory system, throat and mouth. It is commonly used in a tincture to cure mouth ulcers and gum disease. It is also effective in cases of catarrhal conditions and helps to relieve bronchitis, colds and flu. Myrrh is especially effective for restoring the tone and vitality of the skin, and was prized for this in the height of the Egytian civilisation. It is also helpful for fungal conditions such as athlete's foot and is used to help relieve skin conditions such as eczema and psoriasis. It has been found to be helpful to relieve pruritis and thrush.

Myrrh is generally relaxing and can be used to treat stress-related conditions and depression. It has a very mystical energy, and is sometimes used in psychic work and seances. It is an excellent oil to use to assist meditation.

NEROLI (ORANGE BLOSSOM) *(Citrus aurantium)*
Neroli is distilled from the blossoms of the bitter orange tree. The colour of neroli oil is pale yellow and the aroma is clean and floral in type with bitter-sweet undertones.

Methods of use: an essence burner would be ideal but unfortunately neroli is very expensive, so use it in the bath or in a massage or face oil. Neroli is often sold blended with an oil such as jojoba, but this is unsuitable for an essence burner.

Caution: avoid during early pregnancy.

Action: antidepressant, antiseptic, antispasmodic, cicatrising, sedative.

Healing effects: neroli has a profound effect on the nervous system, calming muscle spasms, especially in the heart area. If the condition is due to tension, try neroli as a massage oil or lotion and rub into the chest muscles. Do not attempt to use it to treat a heart condition – seek medical advice.

The euphoric effect of neroli is similar to that of clary sage. It helps strengthen the nerves and is a general tonic. Used in a face oil at night, it will help induce peaceful sleep as well as rejuvenate the skin (especially mature, dry types).

Neroli helps balance mood swings. It can be used to combat a tendency to tearfulness, nervous tension, hypochondria and phobias, and also menopausal and premenstrual tension troubles.

NIAOULI *(Melalaeuca viridiflora)*

Niaouli is closely related to cajeput and tea-tree, all three being part of the *Melalaeuca* group. The oil is extracted from the leaves and twigs and traditionally used for its antiseptic properties. The aroma is warm and camphoraceous.

Methods of use: bath, essence burner, gargle, inhalant, massage oil or lotion.

Caution: avoid during early pregnancy.

Action: analgesic, antifungal, antirheumatic, antiseptic, antispasmodic, antiviral, decongestant, expectorant.

Healing effects: niaouli is a powerful antiseptic and fungicide, and is used to relieve skin problems and infections. It is traditionally used to treat viral infections such as measles, mumps and swollen glands and conditions affecting the respiratory system, such as asthma, bronchitis colds, flu and sinusitis. It is also effective in treating conditions of the urinary tract such as cystitis.

Used in a bath, as a compress or massage oil, niaouli is most helpful in cases of arthritis and rheumatism. It is very effective in sports injuries and general aches and pains caused by strenuous exercise. It has a stimulating effect on the mind and clears muddled thoughts.

ORANGE, SWEET *(Citrus aurantium sinensis)*
The oil of sweet orange was traditionally extracted by expression, but the most popular method is the distillation of the pulped fruit. The benefits are that citrus oils extracted by this method are more widely available, cost effective, and less harmful to the skin than expressed oils. The aroma is like the fruit.

Methods of use: bath, essence burner, massage oil or cream.

Caution: may irritate highly sensitive skin. Avoid on areas of damaged skin. Avoid use if exposed to sun or sunbeds.

Action: antidepressant, anti-inflammatory, antiseptic, digestive, fungicide, sedative, tonic.

Healing effects: provided the skin is not sensitive or damaged, orange oil is rejuvenating to dull lifeless skin. It reduces puffiness and revitalises the general tone. Like other citrus oils, it is effective against oily conditions. It reduces wrinkles and stimulates the circulation. It is very effective in the treatment of children's ailments and will calm and soothe them during illness. Orange is an effective antiseptic, guarding against colds and chills. It is also helpful in cases of fluid retention and PMT, depression, stress, tension, worry and anxiety.

It is said that orange oil helps to bring harmony, balance and well-being between mind, body and spirit. Blended with frankincense, it helps promote a sense of joy.

PATCHOULI *(Pogostemon patchouli)*
Patchouli comes from the leaves of a bushy herb native to the
Far East. It is a member of the *Labiatae* family (which includes
nettles, mints, lavenders and sages). This oil is a dark brownish
yellow, and the aroma can be described as balsamic, sweet,
woody and musty. It is a mysterious oil that some will find a
little medicinal in aroma – you either love it or hate it. Blended
with other oils, patchouli gives depth and body; it goes
particularly well with ylang ylang and sweet orange.

Methods of use: bath, compress, essence burner, massage oil.

Action: antidepressant, diuretic, sedative.

Healing effects: in the 'Swinging Sixties', patchouli was a very
popular perfume; the message of 'flower power' was love
and harmony, and this is exactly what the essential oil of
patchouli imparts. It can stabilise and calm an anguished
state, and is helpful at times of indecision and whenever
dealing with major changes in life.
   Excellent for skin care, especially for dry, cracked skin,
the oil also makes a very soothing massage oil. It can also
help reduce fluid retention.
   *In pregnancy, patchouli may be considered safe to use
after four months.*

PEPPERMINT *(Mentha piperata)*
The oil of peppermint is obtained by steam distillation from the
whole herb. It contains menthol, hence its distinctive smell.

Methods of use: bath, essence burner, massage oil or lotion.

Caution: can induce disturbed sleep or nightmares if used in
large amounts late at night. Avoid during early pregnancy.

Action: analgesic, antiseptic, antispasmodic, expectorant,
hepatic, mental stimulant, nerve tonic.

Healing effects: peppermint is good for the digestive system,
easing nausea, stomach cramps and diarrhoea. It also

relieves period pain and headaches. As an exception to the general rule, the oil can be taken internally – but only a couple of drops, either on sugar or in a cup of warm water.

Peppermint is stimulating and can help with feelings of lethargy, increasing the impetus to get on with things. It can also help release deep fears and suppressed anger that would otherwise affect the liver and spleen.

Like lavender, peppermint is a must for the first aid cupboard as well as for the pleasure of its aroma.

PETITGRAIN *(Citrus aurantium)*
An oil obtained from the leaves and twigs of the bitter orange tree (neroli, see page 95, comes from the blossoms). Originally petitgrain was extracted from the still tiny, unripe fruits, which looked like little grains – hence the name.

The aroma is fresh and green with a hint of neroli.

Methods of use: bath, essence burner, hair rinse, massage oil or lotion.

Action: antidepressant, antiseptic, antispasmodic, cardiac tonic, deodorant, general tonic, sedative.

Healing effects: a tonic for the nervous system, digestive system and skin, petitgrain is similar to neroli, though less sedative and less costly. It alleviates anxiety, nervous exhaustion and stress-related conditions, especially insomnia. Neroli, however, is to be preferred in serious or cases of anxiety.

Some aromatherapists have found that petitgrain helps patients reduce their dependence on tranquillisers.

This oil is a good remedy for flatulence and dyspepsia caused by a so-called 'nervous stomach'. It is also helpful in the treatment of acne and greasy skin conditions.

Petigrain often aids recovery from illness. On the mental and spiritual level, it lifts negative conditions, enabling positive energy to clear the mind of doubt and fear.

PINE, SCOTS *(Pinus sylvestris)*
The oil is extracted from the dry needles of the Scots pine which is a large evergreen tree. The oil of turpentine is extracted from the oleo gum resin found in the wood. It has a strong, fresh aroma, reminiscent of green forests, and fresh Christmas trees.

Methods of use: bath, essence burner, inhalants, massage oil and lotions.

Caution: avoid use if skin type is very sensitive or allergic. Avoid in early pregnancy.

Action: antirheumatic, antiseptic, antiviral, deodorant, diuretic, expectorant, insecticide, rubifacient, stimulant.

Healing effects: because of its strong antiseptic properties, pine has traditionally been used to cleanse and purify. It was used by native American Indians to keep their bedding free from fleas and lice, and it was also used to purify and cleanse their tepees from evil spirits. Pine also cleanses the aura (the energy surrounding all living things) and is sometimes used by healers and psychics for this purpose. It is also widely used for its effectiveness in treating arthritis and rheumatism and skin problems. Pine is also effective as an inhalant to relieve bronchitis, catarrhal conditions, sinusitis and asthma. It will help relieve fatigue and weariness and will work on the energies that help raise self-esteem and general debility. Refreshes tired minds.

ROSE *(Rosa damascena* and *R. centifolia)*
The oil from *Rosa damascena*, the damask rose, comes mainly from Bulgaria. Known as rose otto or attar of roses, the essential oil is now obtained by steam distillation.

The absolute (from solvent extraction) is obtained from the *Rosa centifolia*, notably cultivated in the Grasse area of France and also in Morocco, for perfumery.

Pure Bulgarian rose oil is one of the most expensive oils used in aromatherapy, but it is strong and only a drop or two needs to be used at a time, so it will last a long while. Rose absolute is a deep reddish-brown in colour and thick in consistency (frequently solid at room temperature). Sometimes the essential oil of rose is a dilution of the absolute. Unfortunately, there are a lot of adulterations and synthetic copies on the market. When you smell true rose oil it penetrates your mind and you feel like soaring to the heights of heaven. Rosewater is obtained by distillation. A few reputable companies make a blend of true rose oil in jojoba, which preserves the delicate essential oil, and is ready to use at an affordable price.

Methods of use: essence burner (if you are wealthy). A few drops in the bath is pure joy. For a face oil, buy rose oil blended in jojoba.

Caution: avoid during early pregnancy.

Action: antidepressant, antiseptic, antispasmodic, cicatrising, circulatory stimulant, emmenagogue, hepatic, nerve tonic and sedative.

Healing effects: rose oil is healing for a great many conditions: circulation problems, broken capillaries, varicose veins, arthritis, rheumatism, hormone imbalances, pre-menstrual tension, menstrual and menopausal problems.

Rose oil is excellent for skin care. All skin types benefit, especially the dry, sensitive sort. Skin ailments such as eczema, psoriasis and acne may be improved with rose oil. Pure rosewater is refreshing and soothing as a toner.

This oil also soothes fear, anxiety, feelings of anger, frustration, resentment, jealousy and suspicion. It lifts depression and helps to clarify the mind, leading to positive decisions. In short, it is a wonderful tonic for mind and soul.

ROSEMARY *(Rosmarinus officinalis)*

The rosemary plant is a small evergreen shrub with narrow, leathery, greyish-green leaves and pale violet-blue flowers. It is a member of the *Labiatae* family, which includes the nettles and sages. A native of Mediterranean countries, rosemary has been used in herbal medicine for many centuries. The essential oil is distilled from the leaves and flowering tops. Its colour is pale yellow and its aroma is herbaceous and powerful, like a mixture of lavender and camphor. Rubbing rosemary leaves between the fingers will readily release the aroma.

Rosemary oil is one of the traditional ingredients of eau de Cologne.

Methods of use: bath, compress, essence burner, inhalation, massage oil.

Caution: avoid during pregnancy. Rosemary should also be avoided by epileptics and by people suffering from high blood pressure.

Action: analgesic, antiseptic, antispasmodic, astringent, circulatory stimulant, rubefacient, tonic.

Healing effects: essential oil of rosemary is marvellous to use the day before long, vigorous exercise, as it will help to prevent muscular strain. It has pain-relieving properties. Use it to ease muscular stiffness and aches, arthritis and gout, headaches and neuralgia. Skin problems such as acne, dermatitis and eczema respond well to rosemary. This oil tones the skin and is especially suitable for oily complexions.

Rosemary helps eliminate toxins trapped in the fatty tissues of the body and helps reduce water retention. It is valuable, too, for respiratory problems – colds, bronchitis, sinusitis and asthma – for which steam inhalation is recommended (see page 64).

Rosemary has a stimulating effect on the blood vessels, helping poor circulation, and is a well-known remedy for hair loss. It is also said to stimulate the brain! Certainly it is effective for mental fatigue and poor memory. William Shakespeare wrote: 'There's rosemary, that's for remembrance...' *(Hamlet)*.

SAGE, SPANISH *(Salvia lavendulafolia)*

Spanish sage is a better oil to use for home aromatherapy than common sage *(Salvia officinale)*, because the latter essential oil contains thujone, which some consider to be toxic. The oil of Spanish sage is extracted by distillation of the flowers and leaves of the herb which is native to Spain.

Methods of use: bath, essence burner, massage oil and lotion.

Caution: use in moderation. Avoid use during pregnancy or if epileptic.

Action: analgesic, anticatarrhal, anti-inflammatory, antiseptic, antispasmodic, diuretic, emmenagogue, expectorant, tonic.

Healing effects: for centuries sage has been considered a 'cure-all' and has been used in herbal medicine for all kinds of ailments. The essential oil is very effective as a tonic for the whole system, restoring lost energy. Sage is also widely used to help relieve the symptoms of the menopause, such as hot flushes, fatigue, mood swings and fluid retention. It helps relieve stress, tension and depression and is also used to treat arthritis, rheumatism and general aches and pains and tense muscles due to stress. Sage is stimulating to the mind and helps to dispel lethargy, helping with decision-making.

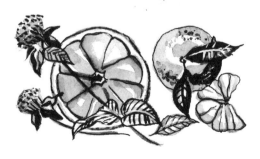

SANDALWOOD *(Santalum album)*

Essential oil of sandalwood is obtained by steam distillation of chippings from the heartwood of a small tree native to India. It has been used from time immemorial as incense and in perfumes. The rich, sweet aroma has woody undertones. It blends well with rose and most other oils.

The trees are usually 30 years old before they are ready for oil production. The best sandalwood comes from Mysore, under strict government control; this maintains a high standard. Cheaper oil is produced from Australian sandalwood (a different species). Its aroma and properties are inferior to those of *S. album*. So-called West Indian sandalwood is a totally different species, producing what is known as amyris oil. This also has an inferior scent, and is sometimes passed off as true sandalwood by unscrupulous suppliers.

One small drop of true sandalwood oil on your wrist will last for at least 24 hours (don't wash!).

Methods of use: bath, compress, essence burner, inhalant, massage oil or lotion.

Action: antidepressant, antiseptic, antispasmodic, aphrodisiac, astringent, cicatrising, expectorant, sedative, tonic.

Healing effects: sandalwood has a beautiful aroma and is an important ingredient in many cosmetics and toiletries (for men as well as women). It has a healing effect on many types of skin problem, especially acne (the oil is both antiseptic and slightly astringent). I have found this oil to be one of the most effective in the treatment of sore throats, bronchitis and urinary infections.

Sandalwood has a remarkable soothing effect on the mind and spirit. It helps calm worries and fears, anger and resentment. It is also reputed to be an aphrodisiac. Blended with ylang ylang, it could help pep up your love-life!

TANGERINE *(Citrus nobilis)*
The oil is extracted from the pulped fruit and smells even more delicious than the fruit itself. Although tangerines and mandarins are very similar and both are sometimes referred to as satsumas, there is a difference between the two oils. The aroma of mandarin is softer, while tangerine has a higher, sharper, stronger note and is very refreshing.

Methods of use: bath, essence burner, massage oil.

Caution: like all citrus oil, tangerine is mildly phototoxic so should be avoided if exposing skin to sunlight or sunbeds.

Action: antiseptic, antispasmodic, digestive, diuretic, sedative, tonic.

Healing effects: tangerine is quite safe to use during pregnancy and is also very acceptable to children. Like mandarin and sweet orange, it is an aroma they know and like, which makes treatment easier. Tangerine is effective in the treatment of oily skin conditions such as acne and congested, spotty skins, which makes this an ideal remedy for teenagers' problem skins.

It relieves fluid retention and can be used to treat cellulite. It is ideal to help ease colic and tummy upsets in young children, as well as being an effective remedy against colds and flu. The mental effect is one of peace and harmony as tangerine is refreshing, uplifting and helps insomnia.

TEA-TREE *(Melaleuca alternifolia)*
The essential oil of tea-tree is obtained by steam distillation from the leaves and twigs of a small tree native to Australia. It has been used by Aborigines for hundreds of years. The aroma can be described as strong, medicinal, harsh, lingering and penetrating. Tea-tree oil has been produced since 1930 from trees cut in the swamps. Because of world demand for this new and exciting oil, young plants are now raised in humid

greenhouse conditions and are set out after about eight weeks in plantations of bushes rather than of trees.

The potential of this oil is enormous. It boosts the immune system and can help a whole range of conditions. Harmless, natural and effective, tea-tree is the antiseptic of the future.

Methods of use: bath, compress, essence burner, inhalant massage oils and lotions, neat application to minor burns or sores. Add to a bland cream or plain live yogurt for thrush.

Caution: irritating only to very sensitive skins. Deep inhalation of the neat oil can cause dizziness.

Action: antifungal, antiseptic, deodorant, mental stimulant.

Healing effects: tea-tree oil has a non-toxic germicidal action and can be used for colds and flu, cuts and bites. It is recommended for bacterial or fungal vaginitis, such as candida (thrush). To soothe burning and itching, which are symptoms of these infections, use tea-tree cream (keep this in the refrigerator if cold application is required).

Elderly people often have bad circulation in their legs; the skin becomes very thin and the slightest scratch can become infected and ulcerated. They will find a tea-tree cream or a blend of tea-tree and almond oil very soothing.

Tea-tree also helps cure dandruff. Add a few drops to your regular shampoo or buy a brand-name tea-tree shampoo. Both shampoo and cream are available from suppliers (for mail-order addresses, see page 218). Sufferers from halitosis and also heavy smokers will find diluted tea-tree helpful as a mouthwash; alternatively, add a few drops of the oil to toothpaste.

Tea-tree has a stimulating effect on the mind and clears a stuffy head. It is also ideal as a first aid remedy for shock and panic.

THYME, COMMON *(Thymus vulgaris)*

Thyme oil is extracted from the leaves and flowers of the common garden herb. The first extraction produces red thyme, which is very strong and considered to be an irritant containing carvacrol and thymol, which are considered to be toxic if used in the crude form. Further distillation or rectification produces white thyme which, if pure and not adulterated (which is quite common), is a safer oil to use. Thyme has a very distinctive and strong medicinal aroma, and has traditionally been used in pharmaceutical preparations such as mouthwashes, gargles, dressings and toiletries. It is also widely used in the food and drink industry.

Methods of use: bath (low dosage), compress, essence burner, inhalant, massage oil (weak dilution).

Caution: avoid during pregnancy. Avoid on sensitive and damaged skin. Avoid if experiencing high blood pressure or epilepsy. Use in moderation.

Action: antirheumatic, antiseptic, antispasmodic, antitoxin, diuretic, emmenagogue, expectorant, fungicide, rubefacient, tonic.

Healing effects: thyme is a very effective remedy for problems affecting the urinary system such as minor infections or inflammation. It has always been a traditional remedy for the relief of arthritis and rheumatism. It is also widely used to treat gum disease and inflammation (diluted and used as a mouthwash), and to ease sore throats (diluted and used as a gargle). I can remember, as a young child, being given glycerine of thymol as a gargle for sore throats. It used to numb my throat for hours. Thyme is also a remedy for aches and paints, arthritis, and rheumatism. It also helps with poor memory and concentration, is reputed to improve the intellect and lifts mental fatigue.

VETIVER *(Vetiveria zizanoides)*

Vetiver is a tall, tufted, aromatic grass with a network of white underground roots from which the oil is extracted. It has a strong woody aroma and is widely used in perfumes.

Methods of use: bath, essence burner, massage oil, cream or lotion.

Caution: avoid during early pregnancy.

Action: antiseptic, antispasmodic, emmenagogue, rubefacient, sedative, stimulant (circulation), tonic.

Healing effects: vetiver is a strong sedative and therefore very relaxing. It works best with orange or tangerine as the aroma of vetiver is very strong and needs to be diluted and blended. It is very effective for stress-related conditions including depression, and is deeply relaxing. The calming and soothing properties of vetiver are most effective when combined with massage.

It is also helpful for arthritis and rheumatism, stiff joints and muscular tension, as it stimulates and warms the blood circulation. It is effective for improving the skin tone and has a gentle effect on minor skin ailments. Vetiver brings practicality to the energies and imparts a strong feeling of well-being.

YLANG YLANG *(Cananga odorata)*

This essential oil is obtained from the beautiful flowers of a tropical tree. The native name means 'flower of flowers'. The blossoms of this tree can be pink, mauve or yellow, but the best oil comes from the yellow sort. The heavy floral aroma has jasmine undertones and is widely used in perfumes.

Methods of use: bath, essence burner, face oil, massage oils and lotions.

Caution: used in excess, it can cause headaches and nausea. In rare cases it can cause an allergic reaction.

Action: antidepressant, antiseptic, aphrodisiac, hypotensive, sedative, tonic.

Healing effects: ylang ylang is sometimes called a poor man's substitute for jasmine. It has a quality of its own, however, and should not be compared unfavourably. I find it helpful for people who are angry and frustrated to the extent of causing physical pain (often medically described as symptoms of unknown origin). This oil can also reduce high blood pressure and calm palpitations.

A blend of ylang ylang with sandalwood and frankincense is very relaxing, easing tension, anxiety and depression. This particular blend is also good for skin problems and oily complexions.

Ylang ylang is a truly sensual oil and reputedly an aphrodisiac.

CHAPTER 8

Massage for Everyone

*M*ASSAGE is one of the oldest forms of treatment. It has a therapeutic effect on the blood and lymph circulation, the nervous system, the respiratory system, and on the muscles and other soft tissues. It encourages the body's ability to heal itself, by restoring free movement to the nutritive fluids. Pressure and stretching push stale fluids away, making room for fresh fluids to take their place. An increased flow of blood increases the supply of oxygen to the tissues.

Massage enables toxins and the breakdown products of inflammation to be more speedily eliminated from the body tissues. Muscles become firmer and more elastic, and skin tone is enhanced with the stimulation of the circulation. The resulting increase of sebum nourishes the skin, and dead cells at the surface are rubbed off, encouraging skin renewal.

The type of massage used today by professional practitioners is mainly Swedish massage, although this does not apply to aromatherapy. Professional aromatherapists study massage techniques in depth. However, the simple soothing massage movements described in this chapter are easy to learn and perfectly suitable for home use.

Massage has a pronounced effect on the psyche. It soothes and calms, creating a feeling of warmth and security. Some people are reminded of babyhood and being held and cherished by their mother. Most babies are continually touched, held and hugged and their bodies rubbed and stroked with oils and creams. Of course the more unfortunate babies, such as the Rumanian orphans, have lacked loving touch and suffered drastic consequences. I'm sure that if everyone received and gave massage regularly we would all be much happier and less aggressive.

Regardless of age, massage can be of help in numerous ailments. In particular, it alleviates tension and fatigue – muscular or mental – aches and pains, strained muscles, stiff joints, arthritis, rheumatism, fibrositis, lumbago (unless very painful), sciatica, headaches, depression, stress and shock.

You don't have to be ailing to enjoy or benefit from massage. If you have treatment on a regular basis, your general health will be greatly improved and maintained.

Generally speaking, in Britain at least, massage is considered a luxury rather than a necessity – a special treat. This attitude is unfortunate as massage is so beneficial. Expense may be a problem, of course. The solution is for one or two members of the family to learn the basic movements, then the whole family can have regular massage.

Family massage improves relationships, bringing you closer together. It could well restore warmth to a marriage that might be failing through lack of touch. Massage is a unique way of communicating without words.

I would recommend taking a beginners' course in basic massage, but if that is not possible there are a number of good books available on the subject. Before you attempt any form of massage, however, there are certain cautions to note.

Do not give massage to someone suffering from any of the following:

- Infectious skin conditions, for example impetigo, boils or abscesses
- Areas where there is an undiagnosed lump or tumour
- Cancer, unless it is terminal and massage is authorised

- Varicose veins
- Phlebitis
- Thrombosis
- Serious heart conditions
- Swollen ankles resulting from kidney or heart conditions
- Heavily bruised or broken skin
- Fever due to infections, recurrent viruses, colds or flu

NB: Special advice on massage during pregnancy is given on pages 130–33, and during labour on page 135.

A Simple Massage Procedure

Let us suppose you wish to massage your partner. Here are some easy-to-follow instructions for a very simple basic massage to relax tension and promote sleep.

First of all, make sure the room is warm and quiet with soft lighting (try candle-light). Choose some soft, soothing music. Take the telephone off the hook and keep the children out of the room until it is their turn. If the weather is cool, keep your partner wrapped in blankets; if it is warm, use a light towel or nothing.

Your partner can either lie on the floor or on a large table. Use a duvet, small mattress or strip of foam underneath for comfort. If you are using the floor and kneeling by your partner's side, use a soft cushion under your knees. If you are more comfortable working in direct line with the back, straddle your partner (this suggestion is only for very good friends!). For just a neck or shoulder problem, your partner may simply sit leaning over a table with arms and head on a pillow.

Beforehand, warm the massage oil by standing the bottle in a bowl of hot water for a minute or two. Always oil your hands first; never pour oil directly on to the body.

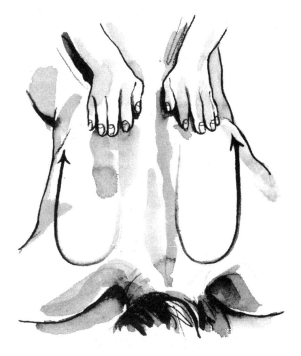

Effleurage

Start by using effleurage (stroking movements). This is done by placing the palms of your hands at the base of the spine, fingers together, keeping your hands loose and relaxed, and push firmly but gently up the whole length of the spine. Put the pressure alongside the spine rather than directly on it. When you reach the root of the neck, glide your hands outwards over the shoulders. Then stroke gently down the outer sides of the back with the fingertips, bringing them to the base of the spine ready to repeat the whole movement. Effleurage will spread the oil and soothe the nerves. Make sure oil is massaged over the whole of the back. This is a wonderfully relaxing movement for both you and your partner.

When you feel confident with effleurage, fan your hands alternately outwards at either side of the spine, returning to the base of the spine each time.

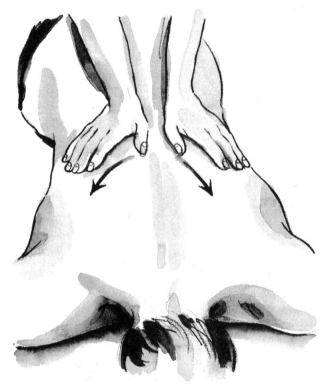

Fanning

To massage tension points at the top of the shoulders, rest your fingers on top of the shoulders (use them as an anchor rather than squeezing the muscle). With the flat pads of your thumbs firmly massage in outward circular movements – left thumb anticlockwise, right thumb clock-wise. Allow your thumbs to be very flexible and cover all the tension areas.

To massage the neck, move your position so that you are facing the neck and head from the side. Place your right hand over the neck and with your fingers and thumbs firmly massage upwards, using forward and then backward circular movement – as if you were looping string, lifting your fingers on the backward movement.

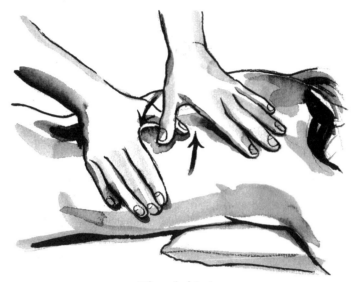

Thumb friction

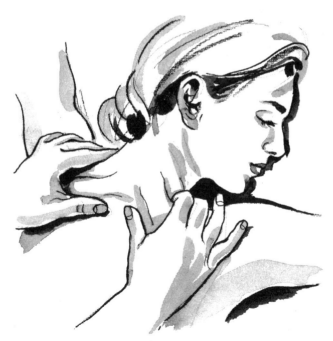

Neck massage

Start the whole process over again, using lots of effleurage movements. Finish your massage with long, stroking movements down the whole length of the spine, using your palms.

When you have finished, cup your hands over the base of the spine to gather heat and relax for a moment. Slowly lift your hands from the back and cover your partner with a towel or blanket. By now you will hear snoring! I would suggest a ten-minute massage to start with, gradually increasing to 15 or 20 minutes when you are more confident.

Head and Face Massage

To relieve tension, headaches, migraine and sinusitis, use the movements below, which are all very easy to perform. Your partner can either lie on the floor or on the bed, with you sitting alongside. Alternatively, he or she can sit on a chair with you standing behind.

For a headache or migraine
Blend four drops each of lavender, lemon and peppermint in an eggcupful of almond oil.

Movement 1: apply the oil to the forehead and face, stroking outwards with the index, middle and third fingers. Begin at the mid-forehead, stroking towards the temples. Then stroke over the cheeks and under the nose.

Movement 2: place your hands together, as in prayer, with the base of the hands resting on the forehead. Now firmly stroke outwards across the forehead with the base of each hand, stroking as you do so with the palms and ending with the fingertips on the temples.

116

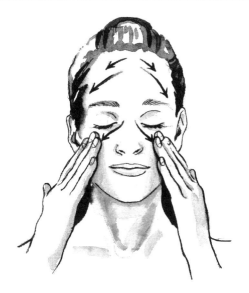

Movement 1

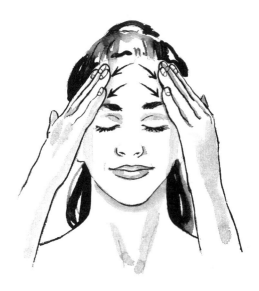

Movement 2

Movement 3: stroke in circles around the temples with the index and middle fingers, as in the diagram.

Repeat the above movements some 10 or 12 times or until relief is obtained.

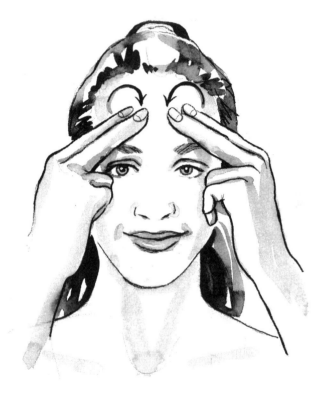

Movement 3

Scalp massage
Using the pads of all the fingers and the thumbs, knead the scalp using firm, slow movements rotating towards the forehead. This stimulates blood flow, relieving tension and pain.

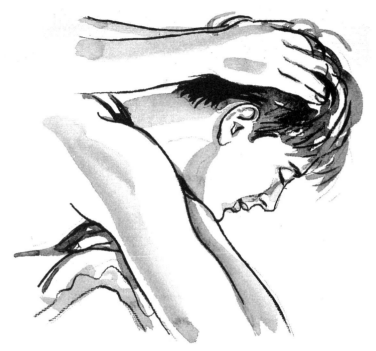

Scalp massage

For sinusitis
Blend four drops each of cedarwood (Virginian), eucalyptus
and geranium in an eggcupful of almond oil.

Apply the oil to the forehead and face using movements 1
and 2 as for headaches (omit movement 3).

Movement 4: using the index and middle fingers, trace a firm
line outwards from the centre of the forehead just above the
eyebrows. This drains the frontal sinuses.

119

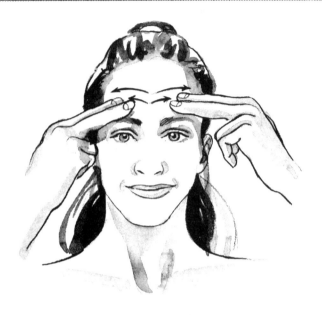

Movement 4

Movement 5: locate the pressure point just inside each eye cavity near the beginning of the brow. Using the middle fingers, press and make rotatory movements around it. This drains the ethmoid sinuses.

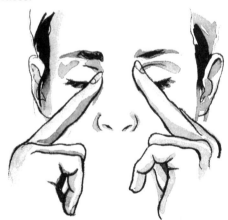

Movement 5

Movement 6: using the index and middle fingers, trace a firm line from the bridge of the nose over the cheek bones. This drains the maxillary sinuses.

Repeat the movements ten or 12 times or until relief is obtained. Include scalp massage to relieve congestion.

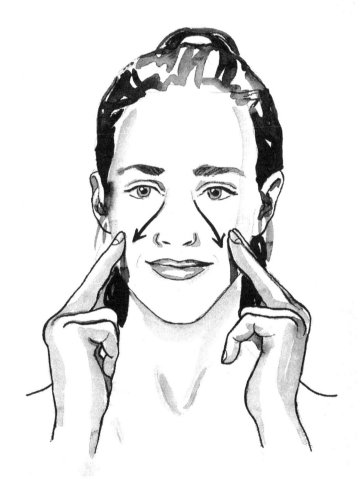

Movement 6

CHAPTER 9

Reflexology and Aromatherapy

*D*ISCOVERED, or – more accurately – rediscovered, and introduced to the West by an American surgeon, Dr William Fitzgerald, reflexology has now become well known as a method of diagnosis and treatment by natural means. It has also proven to be a valuable partner to aromatherapy.

Quite a few books have been written on reflexology (also known as zone therapy), so I won't go into it here at great length. Briefly, reflexology is the use of pressure applied to the feet, both the soles and upper parts. The feet resemble a map of the body, and over the years many different charts have been drawn showing how the zones of the feet link with body systems and major organs.

Reflexologists test each zone (called a reflex point) by using a rotatory movement of the thumb. Health problems show up as tender spots on the reflex points. To correct any imbalance, physical or emotional, massage of the reflex point is carried out.

Reflexology works on the body's energy flow, which sometimes becomes blocked. Imbalances can come about for various reasons, for example bad eating habits. Blockages create overloaded areas, diminishing or increasing energy behind the blockage, rather like a traffic jam. As a result, the body suffers from low energy, possibly headaches and other

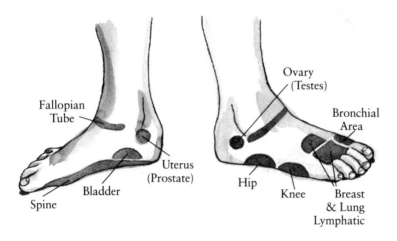

Reflex points of the feet (upper and lateral sides) relating to parts of the body. The points are mirrored on the left foot.

aches and pains, skin problems due to toxicity, and a general slowing-down of vital forces. An excess of energy in the pathways can give rise to inflammation and pain, perhaps leading to more serious, degenerative diseases.

Treating the reflex points helps destroy any energy blocks, thus encouraging the body's own healing capacity to restore harmony and health. The treatment is both relaxing and stimulating; it releases toxins and aids in their elimination.

Reflexology is thought to have originated some 5,000 years ago in China, before the discovery of acupuncture and acupressure (therapies used to correct energy balance in the body). In AD 1017, a Dr Wang Wei was teaching students of acupuncture the use of deep pressure on the soles and sides of the feet, with emphasis on the big toe. The feet were massaged whilst the acupuncture needles were in position, channelling extra energy.

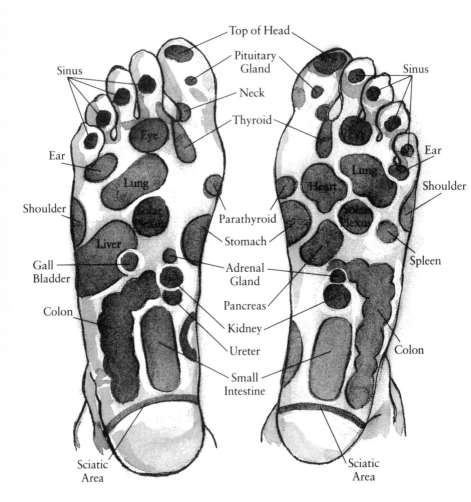

Reflex points of the underside of the feet

Thousands of years ago, before shoes were invented, ancient man felt nature's energies through his feet. The uneven ground stimulated reflex points in the soles as he walked. We all know how painful walking barefoot on a pebble beach can be – but it's a good way of stimulating the pressure points! You can of course massage your own feet, or ask a friend or relative to do it for you.

Professional aromatherapists often use reflexology as a diagnostic aid and include it in their treatment programme. Reflexology massage, in stimulating the energy flow, aids the absorption of essential oils.

Reflexology can be used to treat all kinds of common ailments. Of course it isn't always possible to visit a qualified therapist, but for minor problems there is a self-help method, combining aromatherapy with reflexology.

Self-help Reflexology

A relaxing aromatherapy foot massage

Add eight drops of lavender or cypress oil to a bowl of comfortably warm water and give it a good swish. Take the telephone off the hook, relax and soak your feet for 15 minutes in the warm, aromatic water. Dry your feet and relax on a sofa or bed, supporting your back with pillows. Meanwhile, use your essence burner with your favourite relaxing oil.

Put your right foot on your left thigh. Massage it, using light strokes, alternately up and down. Then, using your favourite massage blend, knead and stroke the foot using deep, soothing movements, alternately. Include the ankle, toes and soles. Stretch and pull the feet upwards and outwards.

Massage the foot for five minutes, making sure the oils have been absorbed. Rub off any excess oil with a towel or tissue.

With a reflexology chart propped up in front of you, press each reflex point of the foot in turn, starting with the top of the big toe. Note any discomfort (you may already be aware of areas that need attention). Concentrate on the tender areas.

When you have finished, place the left foot on the right thigh and follow the same procedure. In reflexology, it is most important to treat both your feet.

Try to set aside some time regularly for your aromatherapy foot massage.

Treating minor ailments

It is possible to treat a specific area of your body with essential oils. (*Caution:* do not attempt to use this method on babies or young children.)

Massage the foot with plain base oil, applying one drop of essential oil to the specific reflex point. For example, you could use frankincense to relax the solar plexus. Here are some further examples:

To relieve a headache: use one drop of lavender and one drop of peppermint on the reflex point on the top of the big toe.

To counteract PMT: use one drop of cypress on the ovary reflex point.

To release anger: use one drop of camomile or rose on the liver reflex point.

Carry out the treatment once or twice a week until improvement is felt.

CHAPTER 10

Pregnancy and Afterwards

AROMATHERAPY is an excellent way for a woman to remain relaxed, calm and healthy during pregnancy and in the weeks just after the birth. At this time you tend to be sensitive and very emotional on account of the hormonal changes and adjustments your body is going through. Throughout these months, you should be treated, and treat yourself, as very special.

While pregnancy may be one of the most exciting times of your life, there can be unpleasant problems, fears and worries to cope with. If you are a first-time mother, you may find adjusting to pregnancy difficult and have to deal with mixed emotions. Emotions are passed on to the developing baby in the womb.

There is always an abundance of good advice regarding sensible foods to eat and vitamins to take. There are warnings about smoking and excessive alcohol intake being dangerous to the growth of the baby. To these warnings one should add that it is very harmful for the foetus to absorb arguments, emotional traumas, shocks, depression, tension and worry. As well as healthy foods and vitamins, the developing child will thrive on love, peace, harmony and relaxation, feelings of warmth and comfort and, most of all, loving communication, not just from you but from the rest of the family as well.

Fatigue is an obstacle to be overcome during pregnancy for, whilst this should be considered as a special time, life still tends to go on in the same old way. Work has to be carried out, the home has to be cleaned, shopping, cooking, washing, ironing done, and the whole household organised. The more fortunate women have housekeepers, daily helps or au pairs to take care of most of the mundane chores. But the average working mum has to cope mostly alone. If there are older children in the family, they can be a great help (sometimes) and of course so can the husband or partner (if so inclined).

Whatever your lifestyle, aromatherapy can help you. You do not have to endure nervous tension. Ask your family and friends to join in with massage (see page 130), or have treatment on a regular basis from a qualified therapist at least once a month (better still once a week). Failing that, there is self-help reflexology (see pages 125–6). All through your pregnancy, as well as having aromatherapy treatments using calming, fortifying and uplifting oils, include relaxation techniques such as meditation.

During pregnancy many irritating health problems can occur. The following are among the most common: backache, constipation, fainting and nausea, insomnia, skin changes, high blood pressure and circulatory problems, such as varicose veins and swollen legs and ankles due to fluid retention. Most of these respond well to aromatherapy. The treatment of common ailments is dealt with in Chapter 13, but for pregnancy there are special instructions and cautions.

When you are pregnant it is especially important to know how to use essential oils properly. You should use fewer drops than generally recommended. Restrict the use of essential oils in the bath or in massage oils to two or three times a week (unless guided by a qualified practitioner). An essence burner can be used every day, however, because it diffuses the oil considerably.

Certain oils should not be used during early pregnancy, particularly those which induce or increase menstrual flow. Although the risk is not great, especially if the mother is strong and healthy and there is no history of miscarriage, I would recommend avoiding all the following in the first few months: cajeput, camomile (including camomile tea), eucalyptus, geranium, ginger, jasmine, lavender, lavandin, lemongrass, melissa, niaouli, peppermint, Scots pine, rose and vetiver.

Some oils should not be used at all during pregnancy: these include cedarwood, pennyroyal and thuja, which are actually abortive and so should NOT be used UNDER ANY CIRCUMSTANCES; basil, clary sage, citronella, coriander, cypress, dill, fennel, frankincense, juniper, marjoram, rosemary, Spanish sage and thyme should also be avoided for the duration of your pregnancy.

If you wish to use aromatherapy at any time whilst you are pregnant, check the cautions on each oil in Chapter 7, consult a qualified aromatherapist and tell your doctor or midwife of your intentions before you start.

Suitable Oils

The oils listed below are considered suitable for the respective stages of pregnancy but use them in the dilutions recommended in the recipes.

For the first four months

The following oils are considered safe: bergamot, grapefruit, lemon, mandarin, orange (sweet), petitgrain, sandalwood, tea-tree, tangerine, ylang ylang.

After four months

Add these to your repertoire: cajeput, eucalyptus, geranium, ginger, jasmine, lemongrass, niaouli, patchouli, rose (in face oil), tea-tree, vetiver.

After seven months

You can include, in low dosage and preferably in an essence burner or face oil: benzoin, camomile, black pepper (not in face oil), ginger, lavender, pine, rose, thyme.

Massage During Pregnancy

To give a relaxation massage to someone in the early months of pregnancy, get her to sit or lean over a table with arms and head on a pillow. Just massage the neck and shoulders. Do not attempt any other massage in the first four months. From the fifth month, massage the shoulders and limbs with the essential oils recommended above. You can also lightly apply oil to the abdomen to prevent stretch marks. During the more advanced stages of pregnancy, concentrate your massage on the shoulders, neck, face and head, limbs, feet and ankles.

Recipes and Treatments

The recipes in this section contain oils that are widely available and not too expensive.

The following dilutions are recommended:

Bath: two to four drops
Massage oil/lotion: four to six drops to 50 ml base
Essence burner: four to six drops.

Throughout pregnancy

Energy blend for massage or bath oil
Two drops of bergamot, two drops of mandarin.

130

Relaxing face and body oil
Two drops each of bergamot, sandalwood and mandarin.

Uplifting massage oil
Two drops each of grapefruit and tangerine.

Bath oils
(Add a cup of milk or one tablespoon vegetable oil.)

Refreshing: two drops of mandarin, two drops of lemon.

Cooling: four drops of grapefruit.

Massage oil/lotion to prevent stretch-marks
Three drops of lemon, three drops of mandarin.

For morning sickness
There is not a lot you can do if you are suffering severely from morning sickness, but the following suggestions may give some relief. Put a few drops of bergamot oil on your pillow or on a pad of cotton wool by your head at night. In the morning, light your essence burner using six drops of lemon. Also try a cup of herbal peppermint tea, or just plain boiled water, with a plain biscuit.

After four months

Relaxing face and body oil
Two drops of patchouli, two drops of jasmine, two drops of lemon. Or three drops of neroli, three of drops bergamot.

Relaxing massage oil
Two drops each of geranium, ylang ylang and patchouli.
Or two drops of tangerine, four drops of sandalwood.

Uplifting/stimulating massage oil
Two drops each of eucalyptus, ginger and sweet orange.

Bath oils
(Add a cup of milk or one tablespoon vegetable oil.)

Relaxing: two drops of bergamot, two drops of ylang ylang.
Or two drops of geranium, two drops of patchouli.
Or two drops of vetiver, two drops of neroli.
Or two drops of mandarin, two drops of vetiver.

For fatigue: two drops of eucalyptus, two drops of grapefruit or tangerine.

For insomnia: two drops of bergamot, two drops of ylang ylang.

Refreshing and cooling (also for headaches): two drops of petitgrain, two drops of lemon.

Backache
For massage oil, blend three drops of niaouli, three drops of ginger or cajeput.

Colds and flu
For use in bath and essence burner: two drops of tea-tree, two drops of lemon or cajeput.

Cystitis
For massage oil, blend three drops of sandalwood, three drops eucalyptus. Apply to the lowest part of the abdomen, over and just above the pubic hair.

Dry skin, psoriasis, eczema
For massage oil/lotion, blend two drops each of ylang ylang and sandalwood, and two drops of patchouli or neroli. If possible, for the base use almond oil with some wheatgerm oil (a good source of vitamin E) added to it.

Insomnia
For massage oil, mix two drops of bergamot, two drops of ylang ylang. Massage the face, the region 5 cm (2 ins) below the breast bone (bra line) and the feet (see Chapter 9 on reflexology). The same combination can be used in the bath or essence burner. Alternatively, try a few drops of patchouli in your essence burner.

To protect against viral infections
For bath or essence burner: four drops of tea-tree or lemon. To protect your home or work environment against infection, regularly vaporise tea-tree oil in an essence burner, and add it to your bathwater if you have been exposed to a virus. German measles (rubella) is specially dangerous if contracted whilst pregnant.

To prevent stretch marks (after five months)
For massage oil/lotion, add two drops each of mandarin, sandalwood and lemon. Massage the sides of your abdomen and the tops of your legs.

Swollen legs and ankles (fluid retention)
For a massage oil, blend two drops each of grapefruit, lemon, and either cajeput or patchouli. Massage using upward movements away from the ankles towards the thighs.

Varicose veins
For a massage oil, blend four drops lemon, two drops geranium.

At the start of and during labour

For fear and anxiety
Use the following blend in an essence burner: three drops each of clary sage and frankincense, and three drops of lavender or camomile.

Compress for during labour
Use two small, soft towels. Lay the compress across the lower abdomen and/or across the vaginal area. To keep the compress warm, use the towels alternately. Add to two pints of warm water 15 drops of any of the following oils, either singly or in combination: cajeput, clary sage, jasmine, lavender.

Not forgetting father

What about father? He needs his share of relaxation during your pregnancy and afterwards.

For anxious father's bath
The first is a 'knock-out' formula, so don't use this if he is needed for emergencies!
Four drops of clary sage, four drops of sandalwood or vetivert, three drops of ylang ylang.
Or four drops of bergamot, four drops of camomile, four drops of geranium.

Father's 'pep up' bath
Mix four drops of peppermint, four drops of eucalyptus, four drops of grapefruit.

During Labour

If you are having your baby at home, it will be easy for you to implement an aromatherapy relaxation programme. If, on the other hand, you are going to have your baby in hospital, then ask the midwife and nurses to allow you to have your essence burner, compresses, massage oils and cassette player in the delivery room.

Perhaps your partner or another member of the family will be with you during labour. If so, get them to massage your shoulders, neck, arms and hands, legs and feet. Lie on your side and have a very gentle soothing rub on your hips and lower back.

Use frankincense or lemongrass in your essence burner. These purify the air and the psychic atmosphere, so your baby will arrive in surroundings free from negative energies.

If you are very nervous, put some clary sage or lavender on your pillow or on a cotton wool pad and waft it under your nose from time to time.

Pain relief

Try the following recipe for a pain-relieving massage oil/lotion: to 50 ml base oil add two drops of camomile or lavender, three drops of cajeput and two drops of peppermint.

Warm compresses can relax the muscles and ease pain very effectively. Have two soft towels or large flannels to use as compresses. To two pints of warm water add 15 drops of clary sage. Soak a towel in this, squeeze it out and place on the lower abdomen. Repeat compresses using alternate towels to keep the tummy warm. For extra pain relief, place lavender or jasmine compresses over the pubic area.

To fortify the mind and spirits, use four drops of either frankincense or lemongrass, or two drops each of sweet orange and vetiver in an essence burner.

One of my clients inhaled clary sage and lavender from a cotton pad during labour. She said the effect was almost tantamount to gas and air. The midwife was most impressed.

After the Birth

Now your baby has arrived, it is still necessary to keep the atmosphere as peaceful and harmonious as possible. He/she will be sensitive to emotional changes and may feel insecure and become fretful.

You have delivered the goods, but your work is only just beginning. Your body has to adjust to getting back to a normal routine and you will need to restore your energy levels – so do keep up your aromatherapy treatments.

Although some women sail through pregnancies and childbirth with little or no emotional change, some suffer dreadfully with post-natal depression. Aromatherapy can be of immense help in this situation.

Do not expose your newborn baby to high doses of essential oils. For the first two weeks, if you want to burn oils for yourself, keep the burner in a separate room.

During the first few weeks you will probably feel rather sensitive. Strong, stimulating oils are not advisable at this time, especially if you are breastfeeding. Use oils such as camomile, cypress, frankincense, geranium, grapefruit, jasmine, lavender, neroli and sandalwood. Keep the number of drops to the minimum, two to four drops in a bath, four to six drops in a massage oil.

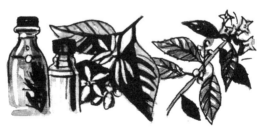

Notes on breast-feeding

As essential oils are absorbed into the body, lactating mothers must not exceed two to three drops for a bath and six to eight drops in 50 ml base oil. Choose from the following: camomile, cedarwood, bergamot, frankincense, geranium, grapefruit, jasmine, mandarin, neroli, rose, sandalwood, ylang ylang.

If using essential oils whilst breast-feeding, remember to drink plenty of water.

To help increase the flow of milk, you could try a massage oil of ten drops of either fennel or dill to 50 ml base oil. Clean the breasts before feeding.

Engorged breasts – try ten drops of geranium in 50 ml base oil.

To restore energy levels

Try this combination: two drops of frankincense, two drops of rosemary.

Post-natal depression

To 50 ml base oil, add four drops of cypress, two drops of sandalwood. (Cypress helps balance hormones.) Massage the abdomen and solar plexus region.

Alternatively you could try the following oils, either in combination or individually: jasmine, clary sage, rose, melissa, sandalwood. Use the oils on your pillow at night, or in an essence burner.

Keep your diet light and free from heavy, spicy foods. Cut down on salt and sugar intake. Eat plenty of fruit and green vegetables and cut out all meat, especially pork – stick to poultry and fish for a while. Take plenty of water, fresh air and some gentle exercise. Try to think positively about your life. You have just given birth to a new human being who needs love, protection and emotional harmony.

Essential Oils for Young Babies

In India, newborn babies are massaged with olive oil. This strengthens their limbs and nourishes the skin. If your baby's skin is dry, massage with almond oil mixed with a little olive oil. To 100 ml of this base oil, add one drop of lavender or Roman camomile.

Mineral oil is not recommended as it is drying to the skin.

Suitable oils for babies
Four weeks up to two months: camomile (Roman), dill, eucalyptus, lavender, neroli, rose (otto).

Over the age of two months: fennel, frankincense, neroli, niaouli, sweet orange, patchouli, petitgrain, rosemary, tangerine, sandalwood and ylang ylang may be added.

Dilutions for babies
One to two months: bath, one drop; massage oil, one drop to 100 ml base oil.

Over two months and up to two years: these amounts can be increased by one drop. (A table of dilutions for babies and children is on page 142.)

Babies should not receive essential oils every day. Two or three times a week is the maximum, whether by essence burner, bath or a massage oil. On the other days, massage your baby with a bland oil, such as almond or apricot.

If you wish to use an essence burner, it must have a deep enough dish to hold water for two hours' vaporising – do not use neat essential oils on a source of heat for young babies. Two drops should be the maximum. Should you not have a suitable essence burner, an alternative would be a bowl of hot water; add two or three drops.

Keep the vaporised oils away from baby's face and head – direct inhalation will prove too much for such a delicate mite.

A relaxing bath for baby

Use one drop of either lavender or Roman camomile. Before adding the essential oil to the water, put in 15 ml almond oil or creamy milk. Swish the water thoroughly. Then add baby!

Colds and snuffles

Place a bowl of hot water near the cot and add one drop of lavender, one drop of eucalyptus or tea-tree. An essence burner could be used if of a suitable type.

Colic

Up to two months: to 100 ml base oil add two drops of dill.
From two months: to 100 ml base oil add two drops of dill and one drop of fennel. Massage the tummy in circular movements, and also massage the back.

Constipation

Up to two months: try a massage oil containing one drop of rosemary and one drop of sweet orange or fennel in 50 ml base oil. Massage the abdomen in a clockwise direction.

Diarrhoea

Over two months: blend one drop of ginger, one drop of orange or camomile and use as a compress. A massage oil can also be made with this blend (add to 50 ml base oil), but apply gently using anticlockwise movements – massage will stimulate the bowel.

Disturbed sleep

To 50 ml base oil add one drop of rose and one drop of camomile or neroli.
Over two months: vaporise one drop of frankincense, or one drop of lavender, one drop of bergamot in a bowl of water or suitable essence burner. For a bath, add one drop each of petitgrain and ylang ylang.

Skin problems (dry patches, rashes)
Up to two months: to 40 ml almond oil add 10 ml virgin olive oil or apricot kernel oil. Then add either one drop of neroli or one drop of German camomile.
Over two months: Make a massage oil consisting of one drop of bergamot and one drop of lavender or patchouli to 50 ml base oil. For a bath, use two drops of sandalwood.

Breathing difficulties/asthma
Up to three or four months: frankincense is marvellous for asthma, as it relaxes the chest muscles and calms anxiety which in turn affects breathing. Also try vaporising lavender and sweet orange. For a massage oil, to 50 ml sweet almond/apricot kernel oil add one drop of lavender, one drop of sweet orange. Massage the chest and back. The same mixture can be added to the bathwater.

As Your Baby Grows

Continue to use aromatic oils as your baby grows. In the following chapter, guidelines and recipes are given for children of all ages.

Relaxing massage oil for babies aged three months and over

To 50 ml sweet almond/apricot oil add one drop of mandarin/tangerine, two drops of rosewood or neroli.
Or two drops of Roman camomile, one drop of mandarin/tangerine or sandalwood.

CHAPTER 11

From Tots to Teens

AT THE end of the last chapter, instructions were given on the use of aromatherapy for young babies. As your children grow, aromatherapy can continue to help with many of their health problems, but of course always obtain medical advice whenever necessary.

Encourage children, especially if they are receiving essential oils regularly, to drink plain still water (bottled or filtered). This not only helps excretion of toxins from the body but removes essential oils from the bloodstream.

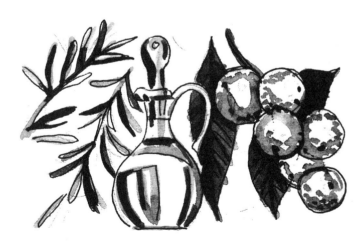

Essential Oils for Children

The following oils are considered suitable for children from six months to ten years (but do a patch test first).

Bergamot, cajeput, camomile, dill, eucalyptus, frankincense, geranium, ginger, jasmine, lavender, lemon, mandarin/tangerine, neroli, sweet orange, patchouli, peppermint, petitgrain, rose, rosemary (in moderation), sandalwood, tea-tree, ylang ylang.

The recommended amount of each essential oil in the recipes given in this chapter is the maximum you should use for a child aged six months to two years (unless otherwise indicated). For older children, increase the number of drops according to the table below.

Essential Oil Quantities Table

Child's age	Bath *Maximum total of drops (first dissolve in milk)*	Massage oil *Maximum total of drops in 50 ml base oil*
1–2 months	1	1
2 months–2 years	2–3	3
2–5 years	3–4	3–5
5–10 years	4–5	5–6
10–15 years	6–8	8–10

Recipes for Children's Common Ailments

Acne

Wash the face at least twice a day – I suggest you use a pure honey-based soap obtainable in health food shops. Rinse very well. Every other day use a gentle facial scrub until the condition begins to clear, then twice a week. Three times a week use a face mask of plain live yogurt (it kills bacteria).

The face should not be steamed as this might spread infection. The same can happen if the spots are touched or squeezed (this damages the tissue and can leave a scar).

When pustules are very bad, use a cotton bud and put neat lavender oil carefully on each one. If they need to be popped, pull the skin on either side of the spot apart using cotton wool pads, rather than squeeze – if the spot is ready to pop, it will release the pus. Apply neat lavender or tea-tree oil to the spot to prevent further infection.

As well as using the scrubs and yogurt, acne can be treated with a lotion: to 50 ml base oil/lotion, add eight drops of tea-tree, five drops of lavender, five drops of lemongrass (if there is an adverse skin reaction use lemon instead). Use this once a day until the condition improves, then every other day. See also pages 153–4.

Asthma

If the child is very sensitive, essential oils may aggravate asthma. More often than not, however, they help enormously, both with opening up the breathing channels and relieving anxiety. To be on the safe side, introduce essential oils slowly and in small doses to start with.

Recommended oils for young children up to eight years are: lavender, sweet orange, eucalyptus, frankincense and tea-tree. For children over eight years of age you may include cajeput, niaouli, lemon, peppermint and pine. Experiment to see which oils suit your child best. Try them in the bath, in an essence burner, or as a massage oil for the chest and back.

Athlete's foot

For children of all ages, use a bland lotion or cream base and to 50 ml add 20 drops of tea-tree oil. A ready-prepared tea-tree cream is obtainable through suppliers. Rub on the affected area before bedtime. Alternatively, dab on neat tea-tree oil with a cotton bud.

A foot bath used regularly will relieve symptoms and prevent reinfection: add 20 drops of tea-tree to a bowl of warm water. Dry the feet thoroughly.

Add tea-tree oil to unperfumed, purified talc and use during the day. You must keep the feet dry and free from perspiration (cotton socks should be worn).

Colds, flu and breathing difficulties

For a massage oil for chest and back: to 50 ml base oil add three drops of tea-tree, two drops of eucalyptus, two drops of lavender.

In the bath: use two drops of tea-tree, two drops of lavender. For essence burner: eucalyptus or niaouli.

When using an essence burner in a child's bedroom, keep it out of reach of inquisitive hands.

Constipation

For a massage oil: to 20 ml base oil add one drop each of fennel, lavender and rosemary. Massage the abdomen gently in a clockwise direction – this follows the natural peristalsis action of the intestines.

Diarrhoea

For a massage oil for tots up to two years: to 50 ml base oil add two drops of camomile and one drop of ginger. For older children, you can also use essential oils such as lavender, lemon and sandalwood. Massage very gently. If the diarrhoea is severe, consult your doctor.

Disturbed sleep
Lavender in an essence burner in the child's bedroom will help. Also try two drops of frankincense in the bathwater, or a massage oil with lavender, rose and/or clary sage.

Headache due to anxiety
Around exam times children are often stressed and anxious. Indeed, the whole atmosphere of the house can be quite strained. Use an essence burner with peppermint, lemon, marjoram and lavender, in equal amounts. The same combination can be used in a bath.

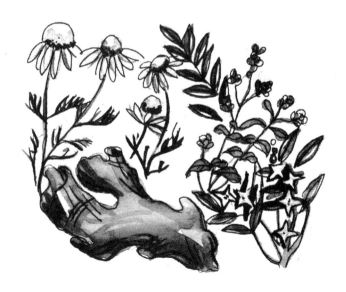

Period pains and irregularities

For many young girls this is a source of much distress every month.

To relieve pain, make up a massage oil consisting of half an eggcupful of almond oil and two drops each of cajeput, camomile, peppermint and clary sage. Massage the lower abdomen with the oil, then give her a comforting hot-water bottle wrapped in a towel to hug against the tummy.

If the pain is really bad, she should sip a cup of hot water containing one drop of peppermint oil.

To help prevent period pains and to regulate an irregular menstrual cycle, try the following massage oil/lotion once a day over the ten days before the period: three drops cypress, three drops lavender and four drops camomile in 50 ml base. (For the adult formula, see page 183.)

Swollen glands

Over the affected area, gently apply an oil, lotion or compress containing three drops of frankincense, three drops of lavender. Repeat three times a day until the condition improves.

Tummy-ache (from anxiety or over-eating)

To 20 ml base oil add one drop of camomile, one drop of ginger, one drop of peppermint. Massage the back and the tummy (in a clockwise direction).

CHAPTER 12

Aromatherapy for Senior Citizens

GROWING old does not automatically mean becoming ill. Learning to be relaxed and to cope with the ageing process depends very much on your mental outlook. If you expect everything will wear out, break down and fall off, then you will not be disappointed – you will have an old age rife with physical problems.

Maybe you have been suffering from a chronic condition and have been told there is no cure. Do not sink into acceptance: take up the challenge and seek a way to improve your situation. Even if you are unable to find a total cure, the change in outlook will at least make the symptoms easier to bear.

People of any age find it difficult to change after they have become set in their ways. But the first thing you must do in advancing years is to stop using the expression 'I am getting old'. Change this to 'I am maturing in the pattern of my youth' (a quote from Dr Stuart Grayson, lecturer and writer).

Learn to relax the reins on the amount of jobs done in a day, and cease worrying about niggling matters – worry does not cure anything. Allow more time for rest and recreation. Embrace this period of your life as something precious and beautiful. Think of all the wisdom you can pass on to those who will welcome your experience.

Nowadays people generally live longer and are more active in old age than ever before. As you get older, you may feel that now your family has grown up and perhaps moved away, you no longer have a purpose in life. Rubbish! You are valuable and needed, and aromatherapy is an area where you can learn to help yourself and your friends. Learn how to use essential oils and, if you are physically active, basic massage skills. Massage your partner, friends, family or neighbours. This can be a very rewarding occupation.

I have taught many people over 60 the fundamentals of aromatherapy and massage, and they have been delighted with their new-found skills. Something special has been added to their lives; they've felt stimulated, too. The learning process brought about changes within their lives they did not think possible. For example, one elderly couple who attended a beginners' class wrote to me to thank me for bringing them much closer together; they felt more relaxed and less irritable with each other.

Aromatherapy can help the elderly in many ways. Use essential oils at home to alleviate aches and pains, arthritic and rheumatic conditions, feelings of loneliness and sadness, depression, respiratory problems, and general tiredness and fatigue.

When using essential oils in the bath, always use a slip mat or side support to prevent accidents.

Essence burners in the house will keep you feeling cheerful and mentally alert. They will also help you to sleep peacefully (but blow out the candle before going to sleep). You can apply essential oils – in massage oils, lotions or compresses – to your painful arthritic joints (if you have any). Whenever you apply body oil or lotion to the feet, remember to wipe off the excess and put slippers on immediately, to avoid slipping on the floor.

Why not run an aromatherapy self-help group in your community? Encourage a communal charge to cover the cost of oils and, perhaps, a massage couch. You will need at least six inexpensive oils to start with (obviously there must be an initial outlay, but you will find the oils last a long time).

148

Elderly couples can help each other with their various problems, massaging each other for aching backs, stiff necks and shoulders, painful knees and ankles. Apart from the relief of pain, this encourages closeness and comfort through touch, which I'm sad to say sometimes becomes neglected over the years. It will bring you closer together. If you live alone, ask one of your children to massage you, or ask a friend to rub your neck and shoulders.

A Regular Routine

If you are fortunate enough to be able to have a massage regularly, either by visiting a masseuse or asking a therapist to visit you, make it one of your regular routines. Massage will certainly help to loosen up your creaky bits, ease your aches and pains, pep up your circulation, stretch and relax your muscles, and soothe the nervous system. It will also help regulate your blood pressure.

If you can employ a mobile therapist, have a group massage session once a week or fortnight. Ask your friends, family or neighbours to come in and share the costs. The more timid ones will then be encouraged to have a go. Make it a social occasion and encourage participation on a regular basis.

After having your first massage, you may feel a little stiff initially, because the stimulation of the circulation releases toxins. Muscles that have not been receiving enough oxygen or fresh blood become sluggish. After the first two massage treatments you will begin to wonder why you waited so long – it is the very best kind of medicine and combined with essential oils will give you a new lease of life.

Some Essential Oils for the Youthfully Matured

(Remember not to use rosemary if suffering from high blood pressure.)

Basil and rosemary: to alleviate mental fatigue (but see above).

Cajeput, eucalyptus and lavender: for arthritis and rheumatic conditions.

Camomile and lavender: to ease aches and pains, muscular spasms and cramp.

Black pepper and juniper: for general aches and pains and muscular stiffness.

Marjoram: for aches and pains, and feelings of loneliness and grief (but not if you suffer from clinical depression).

Rosemary: for bad circulation (but see caution above).

Sandalwood and frankincense: to enhance spirituality.

The recipes below I have found to be very effective for specific conditions. The quantities of essential oils have been kept to the minimum to ensure the safety of delicate skin. But if relief is not obtained, increase the amounts to a maximum of 25 drops per 50 ml base oil. Remember, when making massage oils or lotions, that 50 ml is approximately equivalent to three tablespoons.

For baths, don't forget to add one cup of milk to comfortably warm water before adding the recommended essential oils.

Bath to ease arthritis and rheumatism
Add three drops each of camomile, lavender, marjoram.
Or three drops each of cajeput, eucalyptus, lavender or pine.

Bath for general aches/muscular stiffness
Five drops of lavender, three drops of juniper and rosemary.
Or three drops each of eucalyptus, marjoram and camomile.

Bath for general fatigue
Add three drops each of frankincense, grapefruit and rosemary
(or eucalyptus if you have high blood pressure).

Massage oil/compress for painful arthritic joints
To 50 ml peanut (arachis) oil base (very good for arthritis) add
five drops each of cajeput, camomile and lemon.
If the joints are swollen and inflamed, use the same
combination for a compress. Add the essential oils to one pint
of warm water. Soak a soft flannel or small towel, and apply to
the affected joint. Keep the compress warm.

Massage oil for lower back pain (lumbago)
To 50 ml base oil/lotion add five drops each of black pepper,
lemon and juniper.
Or five drops each of ginger, niaouli and lavender.

Massage oil for general muscular aches and pains
To 50 ml base, preferably peanut (arachis) oil, add five drops of
camomile, five drops of lavender and five drops of either black
pepper, eucalyptus, marjoram or rosemary.

Ulcerated varicose veins
Add 20 drops lavender or tea-tree to 50 ml lotion base.
Alternatively, use 20 drops for a warm compress (see page 63).

For more recipes, see Chapter 13.

Treating Common Ailments and Conditions

THE recommendations in this chapter, for both physical and mental conditions, are for adult use; for pregnant women, young babies and children, see Chapters 10 and 11. Whilst I firmly believe that essential oils are often more effective than orthodox medication for minor ailments and conditions, readers should not endanger themselves or a member of their family by failing to consult a qualified medical practitioner in the event of a serious illness. The suggestions I offer are guidelines only, to help prevent disease, ease unnecessary suffering and support other treatments.

Because each person is different, I recommend several essential oils and usually alternative blends to try – and I hope you will experiment to find the oils that best suit your needs. When making your own blends, choose oils that complement each other (see page 36).

For methods of use (bath, compress, inhalant, etc.), see Chapter 6. Remember to use a 10 ml dropper bottle for measuring out drops.

Unless otherwise stated, proportions given for massage oils/lotions are for 50 ml base.

Measure guide: 1 ml = 30 drops approx.

Conditions and Treatments

ABSCESSES/BOILS

Localised collections of pus forming inflammation and swelling. If large, they will need medical treatment.

Essential oils: cajeput, camomile, lemon, lavender, tea-tree.

Formula for hot compress: five drops each of cajeput, lemon and thyme. Or five drops each of camomile, lavender and tea-tree.

Apply the compress to the affected area twice a day, using up to a maximum 15 drops.

Tooth abscess: as a temporary measure, apply neat lavender or tea-tree with cotton-wool bud. Use an external compress (see page 63). Seek a dentist's advice.

ACNE

Inflammation of the sebaceous glands of the skin, mainly in adolescents. Most commonly it forms on the face, but the chest and back can also be affected (see also pages 143–4).

Essential oils: bergamot, cajeput, camomile (German or Roman), cedarwood, lavender, lemon, lemongrass, rose, sandalwood, tea-tree.

Formula: to 20 ml sweet almond or grapeseed oil, or bland lotion, add four drops each of bergamot, camomile and cedarwood.
Or four drops of lavender, three drops of cajeput, three drops of tea-tree, two drops of lemongrass.

Apply to affected skin daily until improvement. Neat lavender or tea-tree may be applied directly to angry pustules.

Blemishes: to 20 ml base oil, add six drops of rose, six drops of sandalwood.

Apply daily until blemishes fade.

ANGER
Feelings of rage or great annoyance, sometimes suppressed.

Essential oils: Roman camomile, frankincense, clary sage, lavender, peppermint, rose, ylang ylang.

Anger is best dealt with at the time – released, then calmed. If the anger is suppressed, it festers away, causing untold problems. Try to explain how you feel rather than harbour a grudge, then perhaps any misunderstanding will be cleared up. If you cannot deal immediately with your anger, go where you can be alone and scream or, if at home, bash a pillow. Or throw something (preferably unbreakable although this does not provide the same fun or satisfaction). Forgive and let the anger go.

When dealing with suppressed anger, you might find some of the following oils helpful during any meditation or visualisation techniques you may be using.

To bring calm after the storm: blend 4 ml lavender, 2 ml camomile, 2 ml peppermint, 2 ml ylang ylang.
Or 5 ml frankincense, 5 ml rose.

Use six to ten drops in your essence burner or up to ten drops in the bath. The last formula is expensive but worth every penny. If you cannot afford it, buy a pre-blended rose in jojoba oil, add four to six drops of frankincense, and use as a daily face oil.

Alternatively, massage the solar plexus. Reflexology may also be helpful to release anger (see pages 125–6).

ANXIETY
A sense of uneasiness and agitation caused by apprehension or future misfortune; thoughts of impending doom. Excessive worry causing physical symptoms such as shaking, and/or feeling a tight knot or pain in the stomach.

Essential oils: bergamot, camomile, clary sage, frankincense, lavender, lemon, rose, patchouli, petitgrain, sandalwood, thyme, vetiver. Basil and Spanish sage can be used, but sparingly.

To relieve tightness in the stomach area, massage the solar plexus region.

I believe an essence burner and an aromatic bath are the easiest and most effective self-help methods for treating anxiety. In the first four of the formulas below, blend together the undiluted essential oils in a 10 ml dropper bottle. Use six to ten drops in an essence burner and add eight to ten drops in a morning bath or shower two or three times a week.

Formula for working day: 4 ml grapefruit, 2 ml lavender, 2 ml lemon, 2 ml thyme.
Or 5 ml bergamot, 5 ml frankincense.

Formula for rest-days or evening: 4 ml sandalwood, 4 ml ylang ylang, 2 ml clary sage.
Or 4 ml camomile, 3 ml lavender, 3 ml patchouli or vetiver.

Blends to strengthen the nervous system: 5 ml basil, 5 ml bergamot.
Or 5 ml lemon and 5 ml Spanish sage or thyme.

Face oils or lotions: to 10 ml base, add four drops of rose, four drops of sandalwood
Or four drops of petitgrain, four drops of clary sage.

Body oils: add 20–25 drops of one or more of the essential oils suggested above to 50 ml base oil. (If choosing basil or sage, use five drops once a week only.)

When you feel your treatment is working, try a maintenance programme, reducing treatment baths to once a week. Continue to use your essence burner regularly and have massage at least once a month.

ARTHRITIS

Inflammation of a joint or joints, characterised by pain and stiffness. *Osteoarthritis* is a degenerative disease usually affecting older people. Wear-and-tear changes occur in the spine and the bones of the larger joints. *Rheumatoid arthritis* is a chronic disease of uncertain origin. It commonly starts in early adult life, especially in women, and emotional stress often appears to be a factor. The small joints of the fingers and toes are affected, causing swelling and intense pain.

Essential oils for osteoarthritis: black pepper, cajeput, camomile, coriander, eucalyptus, juniper berry, lavender, lemon, marjoram, rose, rosemary. Also, Spanish sage (in moderation).

Massage formula: to 50 ml base oil, add five drops each of cajeput, coriander, lavender and lemon.
Or five drops each of black pepper, camomile and rosemary, and five drops of marjoram or rose.
Or try any of the suggested essential oils singly, using 20 drops to 50 ml base oil.

For baths: try the same blends as suggested for massage. Alternatively, use three drops each of cajeput, camomile, lavender and marjoram, or four drops each of juniper berry, lemon and rosemary. You can use any of the suggested essential oils singly (up to ten drops).

Essential oils for rheumatoid arthritis: as for osteoarthritis. Note, however, cajeput, camomile, lavender and rose are anti-inflammatory and particularly helpful.

Compress for inflamed, swollen joints: to two pints of very
cold water (use some ice cubes), add five drops each of
cajeput and camomile and five drops of lavender or rose.

ASTHMA

A respiratory condition in which the bronchial tubes become
constricted, causing paroxysms of acute breathing difficulty.
Increased secretion also tends to obstruct the air passages,
causing wheezing. Asthma may be due to an allergy or be stress-
related. A predisposition to asthma is often inherited. The
condition is often triggered by anxiety.

Aromatherapy should be used in conjunction with medical
supervision.

Essential oils: bergamot, cajeput, eucalyptus, lavender, lemon,
niaouli, peppermint, pine, thyme, frankincense.

Formula: 3 ml each of eucalyptus, lavender, peppermint.
Or 3 ml each of bergamot, lemon, niaouli.

This blend can be used in an essence burner (six to ten drops),
or as an inhalant (four to five drops). It is important to keep
relaxed if you are asthmatic, so combine relaxing oils with your
treatment. Consult an aromatherapist for regular treatment.

BLOOD PRESSURE, HIGH

In medical terms, hypertension. The blood in the arterial system
always circulates under pressure, but when this is too high
problems can arise. Hypertension is sometimes associated with
anxiety as well as medical conditions such as kidney diseases or
glandular problems. Serious blood pressure conditions should
be medically supervised.

NB: Do not use oil of rosemary or eucalyptus if suffering
from high blood pressure.

Essential oils to reduce high blood pressure: clary sage,
geranium, lavender, melissa, rose, ylang ylang.

Regularly use any of the above oils in an essence burner, singly or in a blend (six to ten drops). Have warm relaxing baths and professional massage or aromatherapy.

Formula for bath/essence burner: 4 ml lavender or rose, 3 ml clary sage, 3 ml ylang ylang. Use up to ten drops in a bath.

Massage formula: to 50 ml base add five drops each of melissa and ylang ylang and five drops of lavender or rose.

BLOOD PRESSURE, LOW
In medical terms, hypotension.

Essential oil to stimulate the blood pressure: rosemary.

To regulate the blood pressure, use five drops of rosemary once or twice a week in a bath (or in an essence burner).

BOILS
See Abscesses (page 153).

BRONCHITIS
Inflammation of the bronchial tubes. Symptoms are breathing difficulties and painful coughing.

Essential oils: basil, benzoin, bergamot, cajeput, cedarwood, eucalyptus, lavender, myrrh, niaouli, peppermint, pine, sandalwood, Spanish sage, tea-tree.

Before treatment, make sure it is not a medical emergency, as can happen in the very young or very old, or someone of an extremely nervous condition or weak constitution. There are lots of essential oils to choose from, and several methods to use.

Massage formula: to 50 ml base oil or lotion add five drops each of eucalyptus, cedarwood, lavender and sandalwood.
Or eight drops each of cedarwood, niaouli and tea-tree.
Or five drops each of bergamot, myrrh, peppermint and pine.
Apply to the chest, throat and back.

Formula for bath, burner or inhalation: 4 ml each of sandalwood and tea-tree, 2 ml pine or Spanish sage.

BRUISING

A discoloration of the skin due to blood escaping from the vessels in the underlying tissues that have become damaged. Some people bruise very easily owing to thin blood vessels.

Essential oils: cajeput, lavender, tea-tree.

The most effective remedy for a bruise is arnica lotion, ointment or homoeopathic tablets, obtainable from health stores. The essential oils listed above are also excellent, easing initial pain and helping to bring out the bruise. Apply any of the suggested oils neat to the injury straight away, then follow with a compress (see page 63).

If you bruise easily, add a blend of five drops cypress and five drops lavender or lemon to your regular bath. This helps strengthen blood vessels.

BURNS

Lesions of the tissue caused by excessive heat. Medically burns are classified in three degrees. First degree burns involve the skin and superficial tissues. Second and third degree burns involve the deeper tissues and bones. Treat only very minor first degree burns. For more serious burns, seek medical advice.

Essential oils: camomile, lavender, rose, rosemary, tea-tree.

The best first aid treatment is to apply neat lavender oil to the burn. You can put the burn under cold water first, but I have found that using neat lavender oil stops the pain very quickly and prevents blistering. If necessary, cover the burn with a sterile gauze and apply neat lavender at hourly intervals, or three times a day.

You can use the other oils listed by adding them to a cold water compress.

CATARRH
Inflammation of a mucous membrane associated with an excess secretion of mucus. Here we are concerned with catarrh affecting the nose and upper respiratory passages. If the catarrh is on the chest, see Bronchitis (page 158).

Essential oils: basil, cedarwood, eucalyptus, fennel, frankincense, lavender, marjoram, myrrh, niaouli, peppermint, pine, sandalwood, tea-tree.

If you suffer from either acute or chronic catarrh, use one or a blend of these in an essence burner or as an inhalant (see page 64) on a regular basis until the condition improves. The following recipes are for an essence burner (six to ten drops) or bath (up to ten drops).

Formula for chronic catarrh: 3 ml basil, 3 ml marjoram, 2 ml cedarwood, 2 ml fennel.

Formula for acute catarrh: 4 ml each of eucalyptus and tea-tree, 2 ml niaouli.

CELLULITE
Fluids and toxins trapped in subcutaneous fat cells, causing a lumpy, puckered, orange-peel look to the skin, mainly on the thighs and hips. The condition appears to be connected with hormone balance, poor circulation or fluid retention.

Essential oils: cypress, fennel, geranium, grapefruit, juniper berry, lavender, lemon, patchouli, rosemary.

Cellulite is notoriously difficult to get rid of. Diet is important. Aromatherapy, using detoxifying oils, has been found to be an effective form of treatment.

Massage formula 1: to 50 ml base add six drops of geranium, six drops of juniper berry, six drops of lemon, four drops of fennel.

Massage formula 2: six drops of lavender, six drops of patchouli, six drops of rosemary, four drops of cypress.

Using formula 1, massage affected areas every day for a month. Stop for four days, then change to formula 2 and start again. During the treatment period, add six drops of juniper berry to your bathwater twice a week and use a rough mitt or brush on the affected areas. Drinking lots of still mineral water is supposed to help. Cut out unnecessary salt, sugar, fats, chocolates and red meat. Eat plenty of fibre-rich foods, green vegetables and fruit.

CIRCULATION, POOR

Sluggish blood flow in the tissues. Blood circulating around the body acts as a transport system for nutrients, oxygen and everything in the processes essential to maintain life. The blood is pumped by the heart which is divided into two halves. The right side collects spent, deoxygenated 'venous' blood from the body and pumps it to the lungs for reoxygenation. The left side of the heart collects the revitalised blood from the lungs and pumps it with force through the arteries to the tissues of the body.

The major arteries and veins connect with smaller and smaller vessels, arterioles and venules. Eventually they become a network of microscopic vessels called capillaries which act as a connecting link between the arterioles and venules. If the circulation is poor, insufficient oxygen gets through to the tissues.

Essential oils: black pepper, coriander, ginger, juniper berry, lavender, lemon, marjoram, rose, rosemary, thyme.

Oils termed rubefacients (for example black pepper, rosemary) stimulate blood flow to localised areas. They cause the capillaries to widen, allowing a greater volume of blood and therefore extra oxygen to get through to the tissues.

The best method of improving general circulation is regular use of essential oils in massage or the bath. The first of the following recipes is a really spicy oil. If you have a sensitive skin, do a patch test first.

Massage oil: to 50 ml base oil add six drops of rosemary, five
drops of bay, five drops of coriander and four drops of
black pepper or ginger.
Or eight drops of lavender, six drops of rose and six drops
of rosemary or thyme.

For a bath: use either of the above combinations, adjusting
quantities, or a single oil, for example ten drops of
rosemary.

COLD SORES

The medical name for cold sores is herpes labialis. They are
clusters of blisters that form on the outer rim of the lips caused
by a viral infection.

Essential oils: lavender, tea-tree.

Use a cotton bud and apply a little neat oil to the cold sore twice
a day until clear.

COLDNESS, EMOTIONAL

Lack of feeling, inability to feel love or compassion.

Essential oils: benzoin, lavender, melissa, rose, rosemary,
ylang ylang.

Use pre-blended rose as a face oil or perfume. Alternatively, use
six to eight drops of rose in the bath.

If you cannot afford rose, try lavender, or a blend of 4 ml
benzoin, 4 ml melissa, 2 ml ylang ylang. Add up to ten drops in
the bath or essence burner.

COLDS AND INFLUENZA

Colds are caused by virus infections of the upper respiratory
tract, characterised by coughing and sneezing. There are some
30 different viruses, called rhinoviruses, that cause colds. There
are others that cause influenza.

The symptoms of a cold are a running nose, 'thick' head and
a general run-down feeling. Some people call a severe cold 'flu',
and indeed a mild attack of influenza may resemble a cold.

When the attack is sudden, with aching in the muscles of the limbs as well as fever, that is true influenza. Typically, the illness is followed by weakness, lack of vitality and sometimes depression. The more severe types of influenza, that sometimes come as epidemics, can be fatal. The greatest risk in these cases is secondary infection of the respiratory tract by bacteria, which is why antibiotics are prescribed by doctors.

Incidentally, antibiotics do not conflict with aromatherapy. Seek medical advice if symptoms are severe.

Essential oils: eucalyptus, lavender, lemon, pine, tea-tree, thyme.

The suggested oils may all be considered prophylactic, that is they help *prevent* the disease. At the first sign of a cold or influenza, have a comfortably hot aromatherapy bath.

Formula for bath: five drops of tea-tree, five drops of lavender. Or five drops of thyme, five drops of lemon.

Use lavender, lemon, tea-tree or thyme in an essence burner (six to ten drops) or as a steam inhalation (four to five drops), either singly or as a blend.

Dissolve a heaped teaspoon of honey in half a cup of hot water and add the juice of a small lemon or half a large one. Drink three or four times a day. Also, take vitamin C tablets.

CONFIDENCE, LACK OF

Having no belief in one's abilities. No self-assurance.

Essential oils: bergamot, cedarwood, frankincense, geranium, jasmine, rose.

Most of us suffer to some extent from lack of confidence, and as a consequence we miss many of life's opportunities. I am not suggesting that merely by using essential oils a long-standing problem like this can be overcome. However, if you are studying for an exam or seeking ways to improve your confidence levels, aromatherapy can help.

I can recommend using pre-blended rose as a face oil or perfume. Try the following blend.

Formula: 3 ml basil, 3 ml cedarwood, 4 ml geranium. Use six to ten drops in an essence burner or six to eight drops in a bath.

CONFUSION

A state of bewilderment or mental disorder; the mind lacks clarity.

Essential oils: basil, cajeput, frankincense, grapefruit, rosemary, Spanish sage, tea-tree.

Confusion is not confined to the elderly – it can happen at any age. Usually it occurs through an inability to relax. When things get on top of you, a state of mild panic sets in causing confusion.

Formula for essence burner: 4 ml Spanish sage, 3 ml basil, 3 ml cajeput or tea-tree.

Use six to ten drops, every day if needed.

Formula for bath: five drops of frankincense, five drops of grapefruit or rosemary.

Use two or three times a week. Once you feel an improvement, maintain balance by using any of the suggested oils regularly in your essence burner or bath at least once a week.

CONSTIPATION

Sluggish action of bowels, which can affect any age group. If toxic matter is not released regularly, debility and depression result.

Essential oils: black pepper, fennel, lavender, marjoram, orange, rosemary.

Massage oil/lotion: to 50 ml base add five drops each of black pepper, fennel, lavender, rosemary.

Massage the abdomen in a clockwise direction, to stimulate intestinal peristalsis (a muscular wave of contraction followed by relaxation). Do this twice a day for a week until regular' movement is restored. If the condition is persistent, consult an aromatherapist or reflexologist.

CRAMP
A very painful involuntary contraction of a muscle.

Essential oils: cajeput, camomile, clary sage, ginger, lavender, lemon, marjoram, rosemary.

Cramp usually comes on during the night or early morning. If you are prone to cramp, a massage oil/lotion used every night may prevent attacks.

Massage formula: to 50 ml base oil add five drops each of cajeput, camomile, lavender and five drops black pepper or marjoram.

During an attack, rub the painful area with the oil/lotion. As soon as possible have a bath – a fairly hot one – adding eight drops of camomile and eight drops of lavender or marjoram. The combination of heat and oils will totally relax the muscles.

CUTS AND GRAZES
See First Aid (page 170).

CYSTITIS
Inflammation of the bladder, either acute or chronic. The symptoms are pain over the lower abdomen and urgent need to pass water.

Essential oils: bergamot, eucalyptus, lavender, sandalwood.

Massage every day in conjunction with baths.

Massage oil: to 50 ml base oil add ten drops of sandalwood, five drops of bergamot, five drops of eucalyptus.

Formula for bath: five drops of bergamot, five drops of lavender.

For pain and irritation apply cold lavender-water compresses. Drink plenty of fluids such as diluted lemon juice, barley water or just plain water.

DEBILITY

Weakness, either physical (due to age or illness) or mental (after a breakdown or trauma).

Essential oils for physical debility: clary sage, cypress, frankincense, ginger, lemon, rosemary, Spanish sage.

Essential oils for mental debility: basil, bergamot, eucalyptus, lavender, peppermint, tea-tree, thyme.

Any kind of treatment for weakness should be gradual. Massage is an excellent way to regain strength, but start with only 15 minutes and then build up to at least an hour. The same applies to self-help reflexology – start with ten minutes on each foot, increasing to 20 minutes.

Formula for physical debility: 4 ml cypress, 2 ml each of clary sage, frankincense, rosemary.

Add up to ten drops in your bath. Relax for just ten minutes. Take this bath twice a day if possible. The same formula can be used in a body oil.

Formula for mental debility: 3 ml basil, 3 ml eucalyptus, 2 ml bergamot, 2 ml tea-tree or thyme.

Use six to ten drops in an essence burner or up to ten drops in a bath until the condition improves.

Formula for mental and physical weakness: 3 ml clary sage, 3 ml frankincense, 2 ml basil or thyme, 2 ml bergamot or rosemary.

Use in essence burner or bath.

DEPRESSION

A low mental condition. It may range from a fed-up feeling to a severe medical condition, perhaps with a suicidal tendency. Despair, feelings of inadequacy, guilt, bereavement, worries, disturbed sleep, hormonal imbalance and illness can all lead to depression. Sometimes a person can be severely depressed without a known cause over a long period. In such a case medical help is required, and also whenever there is abnormal behaviour.

Aromatherapy can be a great help to the depressed. However, marjoram should be avoided by anyone suffering from clinical depression (see Cautionary Notes, pages 51–2). For post-natal depression, see page 137.

Essential oils: bergamot, camomile, clary sage, frankincense, geranium, grapefruit, jasmine, lavender, lemongrass, melissa, neroli, orange, patchouli, rose, sandalwood, Spanish sage, ylang ylang.

Regular use of any of the suggested oils in an essence burner or bath will do much to alleviate feelings of gloom. The more expensive ones – jasmine, neroli and rose – can be bought pre-blended and used as a face oil or perfume. Have regular massage treatments.

Formula: 2 ml each of basil, bergamot, melissa, sandalwood, ylang ylang.
   Or 4 ml grapefruit, 3 ml clary sage, 3 ml geranium or jasmine.

Use six to ten drops in an essence burner daily, or up to ten drops in a bath two or three times a week.

Antidepressant face oil: to 20 ml base oil add five drops each of neroli, orange, petitgrain.

DERMATITIS
See Eczema (page 168).

DIARRHOEA
Loose and frequent evacuation of the bowels. Sometimes caused by a 'bug' or anxiety.

Essential oils: camomile, ginger, lemon, neroli, peppermint, sandalwood.

If due to anxiety: to 25 ml base add five drops of camomile, five drops of peppermint, five drops of sandalwood, five drops of neroli or lavender.
Or ten drops of peppermint, ten drops of camomile or sandalwood.

To avoid overstimulation of the intestines, apply the massage oil/lotion using very gentle movements. Alternatively, use the same combination of essential oils, or a single oil, in a compress. Drink camomile or peppermint herbal tea.

DYSPEPSIA
See Indigestion (page 176).

ECZEMA
Inflammation of the skin characterised by redness, itching, scaling, crusting and sometimes weeping. The condition appears to be associated with allergy and/or stress; sometimes there is a hereditary factor.

Essential oils: bergamot, cajeput, camomile, cedarwood, geranium, juniper berry, lavender, patchouli, rose, sandalwood, tea-tree, ylang ylang.

When dealing with a dry eczema, a massage oil will be helpful. For weepy eczema, try a bland lotion base or a compress.

Formula for dry eczema: to 50 ml base oil add five drops each of bergamot, geranium, sandalwood, five drops of lavender or tea-tree.

Formula for weeping eczema: to 50 ml lotion add ten drops of patchouli, five drops of juniper, five drops of cedarwood or rose.

For a dry eczema bath, use lavender and ylang ylang (up to ten drops in all).

EXHAUSTION
State of fatigue, weakness or collapse due to either physical or emotional causes – all the energies are used up.

Physical
Essential oils: black pepper, frankincense, ginger, grapefruit, rosemary.

Formula: 4 ml frankincense, 3 ml grapefruit, 3 ml ginger or rosemary.

The blend may be used in a massage oil, or in a bath (up to ten drops). Alternatively, for a bath, use ten drops of black pepper.

Mental
Essential oils: basil, lemongrass, rosemary, thyme.

Formula: 4 ml basil, 3 ml lemongrass, 3 ml thyme.

Use six to ten drops in an essence burner or up to ten drops in a bath

General tiredness, including jet lag
Essential oils: frankincense, grapefruit, rosemary.

Formula: to 50 ml base oil add eight drops of grapefruit, six drops of frankincense, six drops of rosemary.

Use up to ten drops in the bath.

FIBROSITIS
Inflammation of fibrous tissue of muscle sheaths.

Essential oils: cajeput, camomile, lavender, lemon, rose, rosemary, tea-tree.

Massage oil/lotion: to 50 ml base oil add five drops each of cajeput, camomile, rosemary and five drops of lavender or lemon.

The areas most prone to fibrositis are the shoulders – very difficult to treat yourself. Ask your partner to massage them, or have professional remedial massage. Alternatively, soak in a fairly hot aromatic bath.

Formula for bath: four drops of camomile, three drops of cajeput, three drops of lavender.

FIRST AID
For serious accidents, seek medical attention.

Bruises: apply neat lavender oil (see page 159).

Burns: apply neat lavender or tea-tree oil (see page 159).

Cuts, grazes: apply neat lavender oil. If necessary, cover with a plaster. You will be amazed and delighted to see how quickly wounds heal using this method.

Fainting: inhale Spanish sage or tea-tree oil, either direct from the bottle or on a tissue or pad.

Insect bites, stings: apply neat lavender, lemon or tea-tree oil. Pull sting out with tweezers if visible.

Shock, panic, hysteria: inhale marjoram, melissa, rose or tea-tree oil, under the nose, either in a bottle or on a pad. Also use an essence burner with six to eight drops of marjoram.

FLUID RETENTION (OEDEMA)

An excess of fluid in the tissues, causing distension and swelling, which may be either localised or affect the whole body. It can come about for a number of different reasons. One of the most common is pre-menstrual tension (see page 183). In pregnancy there is often fluid retention though this is usually quite normal (a protection for the foetus) and nothing to worry about. Localised, temporary swelling occurs in injuries such as sprains. Puffy ankles can come about from standing for long periods (see page 133). Fluid trapped in the fatty tissues is associated with cellulite (see page 160). More generalised fluid retention is often associated with overweight, though it can indicate serious illness, such as kidney, liver or heart disease, which should be under medical supervision.

Diuretics (for example fennel, juniper berry) increase the flow of urine, which can help in fluid retention. They should only be used for short periods and not at all in kidney disease.

Generalised fluid retention
Essential oils: fennel, geranium, grapefruit, juniper berry, lavender, lemon, patchouli, Spanish sage.

Massage oil: to 50 ml base oil add five drops each of fennel, lemon, patchouli, juniper berry or lavender.
Or, ten drops of lemon, five drops of grapefruit, five drops of lavender.

Any of the above recipes can be used in a bath two or three times a week, adjusting the drops up to ten.

FOOT CONDITIONS

Proper care of the feet affects one's general well-being and comfort.

Excessive odour/sweating: regular footbaths will combat this. Add up to ten drops of cypress to a bowl of warm water, soak the feet for 15 minutes and dry thoroughly.

For a massage lotion, to 50 ml base lotion add 20 drops of cypress, five drops of lemon or peppermint.

Verrucas (warts): apply neat lavender, lemon or tea-tree oil to each verruca three times a day until the condition improves.

Tired feet: have a foot bath as above but with five drops each of eucalyptus and peppermint. For athlete's foot, see page 144.

GLANDULAR FEVER

An acute viral disease, mildly contagious; symptoms are swelling of the lymph glands, sore throat, fever and malaise. Medical treatment is required but aromatherapy given in conjunction with it can boost the immune system and aid recovery. The illness can drag on for weeks, with the patient becoming very debilitated and depressed. Massage is not recommended during the acute stage.

Essential oils: bergamot, frankincense, lavender, rosemary, tea-tree, thyme.

Massage lotion/compress for glands: ten drops of frankincense, five drops of lavender, five drops of thyme. Or ten drops of bergamot, ten drops of tea-tree.

Apply the lotion very gently or apply a compress to the areas affected.

Formula for bath: three drops each of frankincense, tea-tree, thyme.

Initially take this bath every other day for two to three weeks. Then maintain the routine two or three times a week until improvement is felt. If feeling very tired, alternate three drops of rosemary with tea-tree. Regular massage and reflexology will help recovery during convalescence.

GOUT

Inflammation and swelling of the hands and feet associated with excessive uric acid levels in the blood.

Essential oils: cajeput, camomile, juniper berry, lavender, lemon, marjoram, rose.

Massage oil: to 50 ml base oil add ten drops of lemon, five drops of cajeput, five drops of marjoram.
Or five drops of juniper berry, five drops of lavender, ten drops of camomile or rose.

If there is considerable pain or inflammation, the above formula can also be used in a cold compress (15 drops) or footbath (ten drops).

Buy pre-blended rose, which can be used on its own or blended with the other oils. Apply to the affected area once or twice a day.

GRIEF/ANGUISH

Misery, intense pain of an emotional or mental nature due to, for example, bereavement, loss of a pet or divorce.

Essential oils: camomile, cypress, jasmine, lavender, marjoram, rose, vetiver.

The above oils will be found comforting. Sniff them in the bottle like smelling salts. After the initial shock, use the oils regularly, either singly or in combination.

Formula: 4 ml camomile, 3 ml lavender, 3 ml marjoram.

Use six to ten drops in your essence burner, up to ten drops in a bath or three to four drops on your pillow at night. Continue treatment for as long as required.

Face oil: to 10 ml base oil/lotion, add eight drops of rose or jasmine, or four drops of each.

Initially use every day, then once or twice a week.

GUILT

Self-reproach. A feeling of having done something wrong or failed to do something that should have been done – happens all the time amongst families!

Essential oils: lavender, myrrh, pine, rose, sandalwood, ylang ylang.

Guilt can be a very destructive emotion. The above oils are a valuable adjunct either to self-help or psychotherapy.

Formula : 3 ml lavender, 3 ml pine, 4 ml myrrh or ylang ylang.

Use six to ten drops in an essence burner or up to ten drops in a bath.

HAEMORRHOIDS (PILES)

Swollen, protruding veins in the region of the anus and lower rectum, often painful and bleeding.

Essential oils: cypress, lavender, lemon.

The most effective method of treating this complaint is to use a bidet or bath.

Bidet formula: three drops of cypress, three drops of lemon.

Swish the water well to disperse the oil. If your skin is very sensitive, add one teaspoon of almond oil or milk. Sit for five to ten minutes. Repeat several times a day if possible.

Soothing lotion: to 50 ml bland lotion add ten drops of cypress, five drops of lavender, five drops of lemon.

Apply twice a day. At night, soak a soft ball of cotton wool in the lotion and place on the affected area (wear protective pants to keep the swab in place).

174

HALITOSIS
Bad breath, generally caused by digestive problems, bad teeth or smoking.

Essential oils: bergamot, fennel, lavender, myrrh, peppermint, tea-tree, thyme.

Mouthwash (ready-to-use): to 100 ml water in a bottle add three drops of bergamot, three drops of lavender, three drops of peppermint, three drops of tea-tree or thyme and (optional) a teaspoon of cheap brandy or vodka. Shake well and use immediately. Make sure you do not swallow.

Mouthwash concentrate: 5 ml cheap brandy or vodka, 5 ml each of bergamot, fennel, lavender, peppermint and 5 ml tea-tree or thyme. Shake well in a bottle and use four or five drops in half a tumbler of warm water once or twice a day.

HEADACHES
Pain in the head usually caused by dilation of the cerebral arteries, muscle contraction or insufficient oxygen. Sinus infection (page 190) and catarrh (page 160) can also cause headaches.

Headaches that are persistent and severe, or have no apparent cause, are a possible sign of a more serious disorder; seek medical advice.

For migraine, see pages 183–4.

Essential oils: basil, cajeput, eucalyptus, lavender, lemon, marjoram, peppermint, rose, rosemary.

Formula: 4 ml peppermint, 3 ml rosemary, 3 ml basil or lemon. Or 4 ml lavender, 3 ml eucalyptus, 3 ml cajeput or marjoram.

Use six to ten drops in an essence burner or up to ten drops in a bath. Alternatively, put a few drops on a cotton pad and inhale. Try a few drops on the pillow at night.

Massage (see pages 116–21) will help to relieve all kinds of headaches, migraine and sinusitis. See also reflexology (page 126).

INDECISION

Inability to make up one's mind about specific issues ranging from moving house to what to wear, causing unnecessary tension. It comes from a fear of being wrong or appearing so to others. Learn to make firm, positive decisions in your life and to trust your intuition. You will then find the problem disappears.

Essential oils: basil, bergamot, coriander, cypress, ginger, grapefruit, myrrh, rosemary.

The above oils, used in combination or singly, can help you develop the capacity for positive, decisive action.

Formula: 3 ml each of basil, bergamot, coriander.
   Or 3 ml cypress, 3 ml myrrh, 3 ml grapefruit or rosemary.

Use six to ten drops in an essence burner regularly. If you have an important decision to make, relax in a bath with up to ten drops of the same formula or any one of the suggested oils. Meditate and the answer will come.

INDIGESTION

Difficulty in digesting food, with pain, heartburn and belching. Food that is too fatty may cause indigestion. Sometimes it is due to tension and anxiety. To avoid ulcers, relax whilst eating.

Essential oils: camomile, coriander, fennel, ginger, peppermint.

Massage oil: to 20 ml base oil add six drops of camomile, six drops of ginger or peppermint.
   Or six drops of coriander, six drops of fennel, four drops peppermint.

If you continually suffer from indigestion, regularly massage the stomach region with any of the above blends and drink fennel or peppermint tea.

For instant relief, add two drops of peppermint oil to a cup of boiled water and sip slowly.

INSOMNIA

Sleeplessness. Difficulty in falling asleep and/or failing to achieve uninterrupted sleep can be a temporary or a long-standing problem. Try hypnotherapy or acupuncture if aromatherapy does not help.

Essential oils: basil, camomile, clary sage, lavender, marjoram, neroli, orange, rose, sandalwood, ylang ylang.

Formula: 4 ml orange, 3 ml lavender, 3 ml sandalwood.
Or 3 ml basil, 3 ml marjoram, 4 ml camomile, neroli or rose.

You might prefer to experiment with different combinations. For example, a blend of equal parts of bergamot and ylang ylang is often effective.

Two hours prior to bedtime: use six to ten drops of one of the suggested blends in your essence burner.

One hour before retiring: have a warm bath with either four drops of clary sage or up to ten drops of lavender.

Try three or four drops of lavender or ylang ylang on your pillow, or neroli or rose face oil. One of my clients drank a wineglass of lettuce juice before bed and found it most effective.

Too much TV can disturb sleep. Resist tea, coffee or cola drinks during the evening – have a cup of herb tea instead.

IRRITABILITY

Over-sensitivity, with difficulty controlling annoyance or anger – being snappy.

Essential oils: camomile, lavender, lemon, mandarin, melissa, rose, rosewood.

Formula: 4 ml lavender, 3 ml mandarin, 3 ml camomile or rose.
Or 3 ml each of melissa, marjoram and rosewood.

Use six to ten drops in an essence burner or up to ten drops in a bath. Have regular massage if possible. Also, try to find an explanation for irritability (dissatisfaction with your life, overwork, PMT), and look for ways to change things.

JEALOUSY

When you wish that you could have something someone else has. Jealousy is a destructive emotion and occasionally so strong it leads to murder. It can also become obsessive.

Essential oils: jasmine, lavender, rose, ylang ylang.

Rose, in my opinion, is the best oil to help jealousy, but if it is unobtainable use any of the other oils. If the problem is obsessive, seek qualified advice. Have massage and reflexology to help balance the emotions and promote self-esteem.

KIDNEY CONDITIONS

The kidneys extract surplus water from the bloodstream, regulate the concentration of salts in the blood and excrete waste products. They also regulate blood pressure. These are all vital processes, so for any kidney condition, such as infections or stones, it is absolutely essential to get prompt medical aid. Some essential oils are kidney tonics, enhancing the filtration of the kidneys.

Essential oils (kidney tonics): clary sage, juniper, lavender.

Kidney tonic massage formula: to 50 ml base oil add ten drops of lavender, ten drops of clary sage or juniper.

Massage back and front between hip bone and lower chest. Use up to ten drops of the blend or any one of the suggested oils in the bath.

LARYNGITIS

Inflammation of the larynx, frequently accompanied by cough, hoarseness or loss of voice and dry sore throat.

Essential oils: benzoin, bergamot, cajeput, Spanish sage, sandalwood, thyme.

Massage formula: to 50 ml base oil add ten drops of cajeput, five drops of sage, five drops of thyme.
Or ten drops of bergamot.

Massage the throat and neck area, from the chin to the breastbone. Do this twice a day until improvement is felt. Also try a gargle with one teaspoon of honey and four drops of cajeput in a cup of warm water.

LETHARGY

A state of lassitude and lack of energy which may be due to a physical condition such as illness, or from a state of mind. If it is the latter and it is serious, counselling may be necessary. But generally a good stimulating massage will do the trick.

Essential oils: cajeput, eucalyptus, ginger, lemongrass, peppermint, rosemary.

Formula: 4 ml ginger, 3 ml eucalyptus, 3 ml peppermint.
Or 4 ml lemongrass, 4 ml rosemary, 3 ml cajeput.

Regularly use six to ten drops in an essence burner and up to ten drops in a bath. After your bath, give your body a very brisk rub with a skin brush or bath mitt. This will stimulate the blood flow and pep up the system.

LIVER CONDITIONS

The liver is the largest gland in the body and is situated in the upper right part of the abdominal cavity, immediately below the diaphragm. It secretes bile, detoxifies poisons and has several other important functions. Serious liver diseases must be medically supervised. However, at times we all feel liverish, perhaps through too much indulgence in alcohol or rich, fatty foods. A number of essential oils stimulate liver function in different ways, such as easing congestion and acting as a tonic (but see cautionary notes, page 50).

Essential oils: camomile, fennel, juniper, lemon, peppermint, rose, rosemary.

Liver congestion massage formula: to 50 ml base oil add six drops each of camomile, fennel, peppermint.

Liver tonic: eight drops of lemon, six drops of juniper, six drops of rose or rosemary.

To improve liver function, massage the liver area with the tonic oil every day for two weeks. Drink camomile or peppermint herbal tea and, every morning, a tablespoonful of fresh lemon juice diluted in warm water. Dandelion coffee is also a good liver tonic.

LONELINESS

A feeling of unhappiness through isolation or not having anyone to communicate with. Loneliness can be felt even in a crowded room, if you are unable join in or feel part of the group. Elderly people sometimes feel abandoned, which can be very distressing. Counselling and aromatherapy may help to relieve the problem.

Use marjoram and/or rose in an essence burner (six to ten drops), or in a bath (up to ten drops). Or use rose in a face oil or perfume.

LUMBAGO

Pain in the low back involving muscles and ligaments.

Essential oils: black pepper, cajeput, camomile, ginger, lavender, lemon, niaouli, rosemary.

It is important to rest and keep the lower back warm. Aromatherapy massage and baths will alleviate the discomfort.

Massage oil: to 50 ml base oil add eight drops each of black pepper, cajeput and lavender.
Or eight drops each of camomile, ginger and lemon.

Apply twice a day.

For bath: up to ten drops of niaouli or rosemary, or five drops of each.
Or five drops each of camomile and lavender.

MEMORY, POOR

Slow recall, often due to mental fatigue and/or poor concentration, or senility.

Essential oils: basil, rosemary, thyme.

Formula: 4 ml rosemary, 3 ml basil, 3 ml thyme.

Use six to ten drops regularly in an essence burner.

The mind should be looked after as well as the body. Crossword puzzles are an excellent way to keep your mind in trim.

MENOPAUSE PROBLEMS

The menopause is the cessation of menstruation. It occurs at a time in a woman's life termed the climacteric or change of life. Usually the process takes place over a year or two and between the ages of 43 and 55. The ovaries at this time cease to produce eggs and the body goes through hormonal changes, particularly oestrogen loss. Although the change of life is a normal process through which all women pass, many will experience quite distressing side effects, such as hot flushes, mood swings, palpitations and insomnia.

By having regular aromatherapy treatments and reflexology, women may well avert some of these unwanted symptoms. However if you are on hormone replacement therapy (HRT), see the cautionary notes on page 50.

Essential oils: camomile, clary sage, cypress, fennel, geranium, jasmine, lavender, neroli, rose, sandalwood, Spanish sage.

Massage formula: to 50 ml base oil add five drops each of clary sage, cypress, fennel and lavender.

Massage the lower abdomen (ovary area) two or three times a week. Also have geranium baths (eight drops) once or twice a week.

Face oil: to 20 ml base oil/lotion add four drops each of jasmine, rose and sandalwood.
Or four drops each of camomile, geranium, lavender.

Use face oil two or three times a week. Pre-blended neroli could also be used.

Massage lotion for hot flushes/night sweats: to 50 ml base lotion add ten drops of cypress, ten drops of Spanish sage.

Massage your feet with the lotion every night before going to bed. Avoid alcohol and spicy foods, drink lots of chilled, still mineral water and take vitamin C tablets.

Formula for depression/mood swings: 4 ml geranium, 3 ml clary sage, 3 ml lavender.
Or 10 ml neroli or petitgrain.

Regularly use six to ten drops in an essence burner or up to ten drops in the bath. If the depression is severe, try a camomile and lavender bath (five drops of each) twice a week. The massage oil recommended for hot flushes is also helpful for depression. Massage over the ovary area.

MENSTRUATION PROBLEMS

Some of the problems that can occur are: *amenorrhoea,* the abnormal absence of the period; *dysmenorrhoea,* period pain; *menorrhagia,* excessive bleeding. The periods may also be scanty and/or irregular.

The massage oils/lotions suggested below for specific problems should be used once or twice a day for ten days prior to your period (50 ml base).

Absence of periods: five drops each of clary sage, fennel, rose and rosemary.

Painful periods: ten drops of cajeput, ten drops of camomile, five drops of peppermint. (Also use during the period.)

Excessive bleeding: ten drops of frankincense, eight drops of cypress, eight drops of lemon.

Irregular periods: ten drops of clary sage, ten drops of cypress, five drops of fennel.

Scanty periods: five drops each of camomile, lavender, rose and rosemary.

Pre-menstrual tension (PMT): five drops of camomile, ten drops of cypress, ten drops of lavender. Reflexology (see page 126) may also help relieve PMT.

MIGRAINE

Recurrent, usually one-sided headache. It may be accompanied by disturbance of vision, nausea, vomiting and prostration.

Essential oils: cajeput, camomile, eucalyptus, lavender, lemon, marjoram, melissa, peppermint, rosemary.

Formula: 4 ml lemon, 3 ml cajeput, 3 ml lavender or melissa.

Use six to ten drops of the blend, or any of the oils suggested, in an essence burner, and up to ten drops in a bath. Alternatively, put a few drops on a cotton pad and inhale, or a few drops on your pillow. See also massage, pages 116–21.

MOUTH ULCERS

A sore on the mucous membrane of the mouth, often occurring when a person is a little run down in health.

Essential oils: myrrh, tea-tree, thyme.

Apply a little neat tea-tree oil directly using a cotton bud. Blot the area before swallowing.

Mouthwash: to a glass of warm water add two drops of myrrh, two drops of thyme.

Use twice a day.

MUSCULAR AILMENTS

The skeletal muscles are subject to damage or malfunction due to injury, overwork, stress and strain. If you over-exercise, the muscles are deprived of oxygenated blood, thereby weakening the fibres and rendering them vulnerable to injury. See also Rheumatism (pages 188–9).

Essential oils: black pepper, cajeput, camomile, clary sage, coriander, eucalyptus, ginger, juniper, lavender, lemon, lemongrass, marjoram, pine, rosemary.

Massage benefits muscles, keeping them free from toxicity and increasing the amount of oxygenated blood to the fibres.

General aches and pains: to 50 ml base, add five drops each of cajeput, eucalyptus, ginger, lavender.
Or five drops each of juniper, lemon, rosemary, and five drops of black pepper or camomile.

Use twice a day for two weeks until improvement is obtained. Then maintain by using two or three times a week, alternating with the bath formula below.

Slack tone: ten drops of rosemary, five drops of black pepper, five drops of lemongrass or lemon.

Spasm/cramp: five drops each of cajeput, camomile, lavender, marjoram.

General stiffness: five drops each of coriander, ginger, juniper, lemon.

Bath formula: four drops of rosemary, three drops of camomile, three drops of marjoram or pine.
Or four drops of lavender, three drops of clary sage, three drops of coriander.

An aromatherapy bath can help relax tired, overworked muscles.

NAUSEA
A feeling of sickness without actually vomiting.

Essential oils: basil, black pepper, fennel, peppermint.

Massage formula: to 50 ml base add ten drops of peppermint, five drops of black pepper, five drops of fennel.

Massage the stomach area twice a day. Use peppermint oil in an essence burner and drink fennel or peppermint herbal tea. For morning sickness, see page 131.

NEGATIVITY
Lacking positive energies or qualities; little or no enthusiam for life; always expecting the worst; hypochondria. See also Anxiety (pages 154–5).

Essential oils: basil, bergamot, clary sage, frankincense, geranium, jasmine, lemon, lemongrass, myrrh, sandalwood.

Formula: 4 ml sandalwood, 3 ml bergamot, 3 ml clary sage or frankincense.
Or 3 ml clary sage, 3 ml lemongrass, 3 ml geranium or jasmine.

Regularly use six to ten drops in an essence burner or up to ten drops in the bath.

NERVOUS TENSION

Too much stress on the nervous system, causing sufferers to be excitable, jumpy or irritable. Mostly affects the highly-strung.

*Essential oils (**calming to the nerves**):* benzoin, bergamot, camomile, cedarwood, clary sage, geranium, jasmine, lavender, mandarin, marjoram, neroli, patchouli, rose, sandalwood, tangerine, ylang ylang.

*Essential oils (**nerve-strengthening**):* basil, bergamot, frankincense, lemon, Spanish sage, thyme.

The best plan is to make a calming formula and add one of the strengthening oils.

Massage formula: to 50 ml base add five drops each of mandarin, sandalwood and ylang ylang and five drops of frankincense.

Formula for bath/essence burner: 3 ml bergamot, 3 ml lavender, 2 ml geranium, 2 ml basil or Spanish sage.

Use up to ten drops in the bath and six to ten drops in your essence burner.

OEDEMA

See Fluid Retention (page 171).

PALPITATIONS

Rapid, forceful beating of the heart of which the person is aware. If persistent, it may be a sign of high blood pressure or a heart problem. Palpitations can also be a side effect of the change of life, or caused by anxiety. If the condition continues and is accompanied by pain or light-headedness, seek medical help.

Essential oils: lavender, melissa, rose, ylang ylang.

Massage formula: to 50 ml base add eight drops of lavender, eight drops of ylang ylang, four drops of melissa or rose.

Apply to heart and solar plexus areas.

Formula for bath: five drops each of lavender, melissa, ylang ylang.

PANIC ATTACKS

Being overwhelmed with terror for no apparent reason. The condition can come on at any time, often with gasping, rapid breathing.

Essential oils: basil, clary sage, frankincense, lavender, rose, tea-tree, vetiver.

Formula for preventing attacks: to 50 ml base add ten drops frankincense, ten drops of lavender or rose.
Or add a few drops of clary sage to pre-blended rose oil.

At onset of an attack: waft a bottle of frankincense, lavender or tea-tree under the nose like smelling salts. Do not inhale too deeply, however, as you may feel dizzy.

In addition to aromatherapy treatment, massage the solar plexus area.

PHLEBITIS

Inflammation of a vein, usually affecting a leg. Characteristic symptoms are swelling, pain and tenderness. The leg looks white and feels heavy.

Essential oils: camomile, lavender, lemon.

Phlebitis should not be massaged. Make a cold compress using the above oils, or add them to a warm bath.

PREMENSTRUAL TENSION (PMT)

See Menstruation Problems (page 183).

PSORIASIS

A non-infective chronic skin disease characterised by dry, scaly, red areas, most commonly in the flexure area of elbows, knees and wrists.

The cause is unknown, though worry and stress are predisposing factors. Aromatherapy treatment of this intractable condition is mainly aimed at quelling anxiety and stress and stimulating the growth of new skin cells to replace the damaged ones.

Essential oils: bergamot, cajeput, camomile, cedarwood, geranium, lavender, rose, sandalwood.

Lotion: to 50 ml base, add eight drops each of bergamot, cajeput and geranium.
Or five drops each of camomile, lavender, sandalwood, five drops of cedarwood or rose.

Apply twice a day until there is an improvement, then once a day. Maintain improvement using the lotion twice a week. If the condition flares up again, increase the application until it subsides. Try different combinations if no marked improvement is seen.

Also add a few drops of lavender or sandalwood to your bath.

RHEUMATISM

In medical terminology, rheumatism embraces a whole range of disorders involving painful muscles and joints, including rheumatoid arthritis and osteoarthritis. In general usage, however, rheumatism is confined to conditions where the pain is mainly in the muscles rather than the joint itself. This is the kind of rheumatism that principally concerns us here. It often occurs after getting getting cold and wet, in damp weather, from being in a draught, etc.

Aromatherapy treatment concentrates on eliminating toxins, stimulating the circulation, and easing pain and muscle stiffness.

Essential oils: black pepper, cajeput, camomile, eucalyptus, lavender, lemon, marjoram, rosemary, Spanish sage, thyme.

Massage formula: to 50 ml base add eight drops of lemon, eight drops of rosemary, eight drops of cajeput or eucalyptus.
Or eight drops of camomile, eight drops of lavender, eight drops of marjoram or Spanish sage.

To ease rheumatism, it is a good idea to have regular massage. Also use the above combinations or any of the suggested oils in a bath (up to ten drops).

SEXUAL RESPONSE, LOW

The problem is usually psychological and may need professional help. Anxiety is a frequent cause of frigidity or impotence. Physical disorders, such as diabetes, may affect sexual response so do seek medical advice.

Essential oils: cedarwood, clary sage, fennel, jasmine, rosemary, sandalwood, ylang ylang.

To arouse sexual response in your partner, massage the erogenous zones with light, stroking movements using a blend of essential oils reputed to be aphrodisiacs. If impotence or frigidity does not respond, seek qualified counselling.

Lovers' blend: to 30 ml base add five drops of sandalwood, five drops of ylang ylang, three drops of fennel, two drops of clary sage.

SINUSITIS

Inflammation of an air sinus – a bony cavity in the skull. There is one on each side of the nose (the maxillary sinuses), and two at the root of the nose in the frontal bone (the frontal sinuses). Like the nose, they are lined with mucous membrane.

The symptoms of sinusitis include pain in the forehead or around the eyes, nasal congestion and headache. Acute sinusitis may follow a cold and the patient suffers from a severe headache – prompt medical supervision should be sought. In chronic sinusitis, the pain is duller, and there is constant mucous discharge in the nose that may be caused by allergy.

Essential oils: cedarwood, lemon, eucalyptus, geranium, lavender, niaouli, peppermint, pine.

Formula: 3 ml cedarwood, 3 ml lemon, 2 ml niaouli, 2 ml lavender.
Or 3 ml geranium, 3 ml niaouli, 2 ml eucalyptus, 2 ml peppermint.

Either of the above combinations can be used in steam inhalation (see page 64). To prevent sinusitis, use any of the suggested oils or blends in your essence burner.

SORE THROATS

Soreness and swelling of the throat due to infection (colds, flu), smoking or a dusty atmosphere.

Essential oils: bergamot, cajeput, lavender, lemon, geranium, tea-tree, thyme.

The same essential oils are recommended for tonsillitis.

Massage formula for throat area: to 50 ml base add eight drops each of bergamot, lavender, tea-tree or thyme.

Gargle: to a cup of warm water add one teaspoon of honey and two drops each of lavender, lemon, tea-tree. Stir well, gargle in the usual way (do not swallow).

SPRAINS
See pages 63–4.

STRESS AND STRAIN
Over-exertion, mental and physical, where all the resources are taxed.

Essential oils: basil, bergamot, frankincense, neroli,
    ylang ylang.

Relaxation is not the only requirement in this situation. Learn how to avoid taking on too much! (Also see Chapter 15.)

Formula: 3 ml bergamot, 3 ml frankincense, 2 ml basil,
    2 ml neroli or ylang ylang.

Regularly use six to ten drops in an essence burner or up to ten drops in a bath. Have regular massage.

SUNBURN
Sore red patches on the skin as a result of having spent too much time in the hot sunshine. Fair-skinned people are particularly susceptible.

Essential oils: bergamot, camomile, lavender, sandalwood.

In the event of sunburn, apply neat lavender to the affected part. This will ease pain and prevent blistering.

Do not use bergamot just prior to or during sunbathing as it is one of the oils that are classed as phototoxic. It is safe to use afterwards, however, and is effective used in an after-sun oil or lotion.

After-sun soothing oil/lotion: to 50 ml base, add six drops of
    bergamot, six drops of lavender, five drops of camomile,
    five drops of sandalwood.

TEARFULNESS

Proneness to tears for no apparent reason, though often linked with PMT and the menopause.

Essential oils: cypress, geranium, lavender, marjoram, neroli.

Formula: 3 ml lavender, 3 ml marjoram, 2 ml cypress,
2 ml neroli or geranium.

Use six to ten drops in an essence burner or up to ten drops in a bath. A neroli face oil at night or used as a perfume will also help.

TONSILLITIS

Inflammation of the tonsils, lymphoid tissue at the back of the throat.

Treatment is as recommended for Sore Throats (see page 190).

THRUSH

Infection of mucous membrane by the fungus *Candida albicans*. The vagina is most commonly affected.

Essential oils: lemon, geranium, tea-tree.

Formula for vaginal swab: to a cup of warm water add two
drops each of lemon and tea-tree oil.

With a cotton wool pad, swab just inside the vagina. Alternatively, use the same formula to bathe the affected area in a bidet, using four to five drops and swishing the water well.

Plain live yoghurt is a well known and successful remedy for thrush. Eat the yoghurt on an empty stomach so its assimilation is fast. The yoghurt may also be used on a swab. A good method is to soak a tampon or cotton wool ball in a teaspoon of yoghurt plus two drops of tea-tree oil. Put the tampon just inside the vagina before going to bed and leave it overnight.

Ready-made tea-tree cream can be purchased. Keep it in the fridge so that it is nice and cold on application to the vagina.

TOOTHACHE

Pain, either dull or acute, from a decayed tooth, often radiating to the face.

Essential oils: cajeput, lavender, tea-tree.

To relieve the pain before getting to a dentist, use a small amount of any of the above oils neat on the painful tooth.

VARICOSE VEINS

Dilated veins, in particular in the legs, due to loss of elasticity in the vessel walls and valves so that the blood flow becomes inefficient. The condition causes aching and tiredness in the limbs. Ulceration can occur.

Essential oils: cypress, lemon.

Never massage below the varicosity, as this will cause more swelling of the vein. Light, upward strokes from the affected area are helpful, however. Do not massage too deeply.

Lotion: to 50 ml base add ten drops of cypress, ten drops of lemon.

Lightly stroke the affected area twice a day. Whenever possible the limbs should be rested in an elevated position (above waist level).

For varicose ulcers: use 15–20 drops of tea-tree in a cold compress. Add the same number of drops to 50 ml base oil or lotion.

Pure honey is also a good healing agent. Apply the purest honey to the ulcer and cover with a lint dressing. Change and reapply dressings frequently. Drink plenty of camomile tea to aid healing.

WRINKLES

Creasing of the skin as it gets older, particularly noticeable on the face. The wrinkling is caused by the underlying support, that is collagen connective tissue, diminishing.

Essential oils: frankincense, lemon, orange, tangerine.

Massage oil/lotion: to 50 ml base add 15 drops of lemon, ten
   drops of frankincense.

When using the oil or lotion on the face, avoid the delicate eye area. Use regularly, at least once or twice a week.

CHAPTER 14

The Holistic Approach and Emotional Healing

*T*HE holistic approach to healing covers all the dimensions of mind, body, spirit and emotions. Our health concerns more than just our physical body and so attention must be paid to the way we feel emotionally as well as to the way we feel and perform physically. Things that adversely affect us both emotionally and mentally will manifest in the body as physical symptoms, illness and eventually disease; physical fitness alone is not enough. Emotional healing starts with being happy, something that is not always easily explained as it means different things to different people. For some, happiness comes from outside themselves, in the shape of people, pleasure, spending money, work, and holidays. Others feel that the trappings of wealth and the regard of other people mean nothing if you have not got peace of mind and do not feel good about yourself. Whatever your style, true happiness is an inner feeling of peace, tranquillity and joy that is experienced at just being who you are, where you are, no matter why you are.

Emotions that create feelings are triggered by responses in the part of the brain referred to as the limbic system, which is the part of the primitive brain responsible for the basic emotions and needs of the human being, for example, hunger, thirst and sexual appetite. The limbic system is linked with the endocrine gland system and the secretion of hormones. The release of neurochemicals and hormones into the bloodstream responds to strong emotional feelings such as love, hate, fear and anger. This affects the feelings, responses and performance of the physical body. Because an emotion is the primary motivation to how our bodies respond, for example by kissing or kicking, the emotion is completed and released. If the situation surrounding the emotion is not completed, for example when the feeling of love or anger is suppressed, it remains trapped within the cells of the body.

If layer after layer of emotions and feelings are continually suppressed and repressed, eventually the parts of the body most likely to be affected will respond in an effort to be released. This can result in the related area of the physical body manifesting symptoms. For example:

- Anger and resentment affects the liver and gall bladder
- Fear and anxiety affects the stomach and bowels
- Trauma and unhappiness in childhood affects the kidneys
- Fear of rejection affects the sexual organs
- Fear of life and responsibility affects the lungs
- Fear of expressing creativity affects the reproductive system
- Lack of joy and love affects the heart and circulation
- Tension and worry affects the muscular system
- Belief in struggle and lack of fun affects the pancreas and heart
- Fear of moving forward affects the hips, knees and feet
- Fear of saying what you need to say affects the throat
- Too much going on in your life affects the head, sinuses and immune system
- Criticism, both of self and of others, affects the balance of cell-regeneration

Aromatherapy is based on creating complete harmony of all the energies, and certain essential oils are very effective in helping to release emotional toxins.

Try the following blends to help gently release congestion and soothe the flow of energy.

Methods of use: burner, massage oils (30 ml base oil) or bath (six to eight drops). Before using any of the suggested oils, check cautionary notes if you have a medical condition, epileptic or pregnant.

Anger and resentment
Four drops each of peppermint, lemon, Roman camomile (if you suffer with liver disease or have undergone a transplant, refer to page 50).

Fear and anxiety
Four drops each of bergamot, clary sage, ginger.

Childhood unhappiness
Four drops each of lavender, clary sage, sweet orange.

Rejection
Four drops each of jasmine, sandalwood, coriander.

Life and responsibility
Three drops each of frankincense, geranium, benzoin, lavandin.

Fear of creativity
Four drops each of cypress, Spanish or clary sage, melissa.

Lack of love and joy
Four drops each of rose, ylang ylang, sandalwood.

Tension (muscular)
Four drops each of lavender, marjoram, camomile.

Tension (mental)
Four drops each of basil, grapefruit, sandalwood.

Struggle and lack of fun
Four drops each of eucalyptus, lemon, ginger.

Inability to move forward in life
Four drops each of frankincense, cedarwood (Atlas), marjoram.

Fear of speaking up
Four drops each of bergamot, ylang ylang, rose.

Too much going on
Three drops each of geranium, cedarwood (Virginian), lemon, pine.

Criticism of self and others
Four drops each of grapefruit, ylang ylang, coriander.

Healing our emotions is not an easy task as we are not always aware of the root causes, and mostly push them aside to get on with our lives. If you are determined to make positive changes, here are a few ideas to help.

On how to be unhappy

- If you are over-stressed and tired, ignore it and keep pushing yourself.
- If you choose to do things that are considered bad for you, feel guilty about them.
- Do the things you don't like and avoid doing what you really want.
- Be resentful and hypercritical, especially towards yourself.

- Avoid making any changes which could bring you greater satisfaction and joy.
- Be depressed, self-pitying, envious and angry, blame everyone and everything for things that are wrong in your life.
- Cultivate the experience of your life as meaningless and of little value.

On how to become happy

- Do things that bring a sense of fulfilment, joy and purpose, and validate your worth.
- See your life as your own creation and strive to make it a positive one.
- Pay close and loving attention to yourself, tuning into your needs on all levels.
- Release all negative emotions, resentment, envy, fear, sadness and anger.
- Express your feelings appropriately; don't hold on. Forgive yourself.
- Love yourself and everyone else. See love as your main purpose and expression in your life.
- Create fun-loving, honest relationships. Try to heal old wounds in relationships, perhaps with parents or partners.
- Accept yourself and everything in your life as an opportunity for growth and learning.
- If you mess up, forgive yourself, learn from the experience and move on.
- Keep a sense of humour.

Aromatherapy can help bring about changes in your emotional well-being by helping the mind relax and be calm. Decisions and change cannot be made when the mind is troubled. Having a regular massage works on the physical body to help gently release stored and repressed emotions. I have treated many clients who have simply burst into tears half-way through a massage whilst experiencing a release of negative emotions. Because massage works on the subtle energies, this is an excellent way of dealing with emotional release.

Not all of our emotional responses are suppressed or buried; they can change from day to day, and can therefore be treated as and when they appear. The following list offers a few ideas to help emotional situations.

Use in an essence burner for quicker and more instant effect. Choose any one oil from the suggestions or a combination of three, maximum four, oils, or inhale oils from a cotton wool pad. Before using any of the oils check against cautions if you have a medical condition, such as epilepsy, or are pregnant.

General stress and anxiety
Bergamot, clary sage, jasmine, lavender, rose, sandalwood, ylang ylang. Try a combination of bergamot, jasmine and sandalwood for a total 'de-stress' formula.
(See details on stress management in Chapter 15.)

Fear
Of coming events: camomile (Roman), clary sage,　fennel, jasmine, sandalwood.
Of people: basil, lavender, ylang ylang.
Of failure: frankincense, geranium.
Of interviews: grapefruit, jasmine, rose.
Of attack: camomile (Roman), clary sage, frankincense.
Of letting go: bergamot, frankincence, grapefruit, rose.
Of change: lavender, frankincense, orange (sweet), ylang ylang.

Anger
Basil, bergamot, camomile, cedarwood, clary sage, lavender, patchouli, petitgrain, rose, vetiver.

Sadness
Melissa, myrrh, orange (sweet), rose, tangerine.

Guilt
Clary sage, jasmine, lavender, marjoram, myrrh, pine, rose, sandalwood, vetiver, ylang ylang.

Feeling inadequate
Basil, cedarwood, coriander, geranium, fennel, frankincense, ylang ylang.

Envy and jealousy
Basil, jasmine, lavender, rose, ylang ylang.

Feeling selfish
Camomile (Roman), cypress, lavender, neroli, rose.

Low self-esteem
Camomile (Roman), cedarwood (Atlas), geranium, juniper berry, neroli, sandalwood.

Monday morning feeling
Basil, lemon, lemongrass, rosemary.

Lethargy
Cajeput, eucalyptus, grapefruit, rosemary.

Irritability
Bergamot, camomile (Roman), clary sage, neroli, patchouli, rose, sandalwood, ylang ylang.

Procrastination
Cajeput, eucalpytus, frankincense, grapefruit.

Confidence

Frankincense, geranium, jasmine, rose.

If emotional problems are deep seated and traumatic, it would be wise to seek qualified help before considering tackling any problems. If you feel confident in self-help, there are some suggested books on pages 217–8.

Aromatherapy will help to bring about a calmer and more peaceful approach to life, helping to change attitudes, behaviour and feelings.

CHAPTER 15

Stress Management

*S*TRESS is the epidemic of the twentieth century, and the word stress is used to describe many emotional and physical symptoms. Buzz words, such as burn-out, overload, underload and conflict, all describe conditions and situations that most people find themselves in at some time in their life. Stress has many causes and manifests itself in many different ways, and I believe we are only just discovering just how seriously it affects our lives. However, everything must be put in perspective and there are many situations and events that cannot be answered purely from a stress management point of view.

What does the word stress mean? It is a contraction of the word distress, which means mental pain and anguish. Stress is related to all three of the dimensions of human experience, mental, physical and emotional. Under stress there is an emphasis or urgency which is classed as strain.

The human stress response is quite normal, and is triggered by fear. It is called the 'fight or flight syndrome' which automatically clicks in when we are faced with danger, or we think we are in danger. The adrenal glands, which are situated on top of the kidneys, secrete adrenaline, a hormone responsible for increasing our heart rate, blood pressure, blood sugar and blood fats. Adrenaline also makes us sweat to cool down the body which gets very hot as it prepares itself for battle. Our pupils dilate, and our muscles become tense. If you ever took part in school races, think of how you felt at the start line, waiting for the race to begin. The stress response also affects the stomach and abdomen and causes an imbalance in the need to urinate or defecate. The feeling of 'butterflies' in the stomach is a response to nervousness or excitement which can be pleasant or unpleasant.

The production of extra adrenaline is not wholly dangerous: on the contrary, we need this response to achieve goals and deadlines, and in many instances people do work better under pressure. To this end stress can be helpful rather than harmful, and it is important not to see stress as our all-time enemy. The harm is done when we can no longer differentiate between the stressed state and the normal state. This occurs when we are unable to 'switch off', and continue to produce an excess of adrenaline, keeping our minds and bodies on 'red alert'. When this state becomes almost permanent, we then suffer with physical and mental symptoms caused by too much adrenaline, and we slip into a tired acceptance of coping.

In the seventies and eighties, the expression 'burn-out' was more widely associated with the whizz-kid dealers of the City's money markets. They lived on the adrenaline rush, brought about by the excitement and stimulation of the job. Working at optimum performance all day meant many were unable to relax after work, and for some this meant high alcohol consumption, drugs and late nights. After a relatively short period of time the dealers, some as young as 27, were considered to be finished, burnt out, and this still goes on. One of my clients was very worried about her husband, who was a dealer. He was showing the classic signs of stress, and she was concerned that he would suffer the consquences of 'burn-out'. We discussed how she could help relieve his stress levels, and she decided to come on one of my massage courses. She bought a couch and some clary sage, frankincense and lavender oil and gave him a massage at least three times a week. He benefited enormously.

Stress occurs through our perception of the world around us: if we see things in a negative way, this will create a stressful response in us. Hans Seyles wrote: 'It is not the stressors (the causes of stress) that are harmful to us, but the way we respond to them'. Learning new perceptions and responses is another matter and not so simple to do. How we see things in life mainly comes from how we were brought up. The cultures and environments that we experienced as babies and children have formed how we see things as adults. The needs of the community are nowadays not so important to the individual and we are seeing perhaps that the framework of the family unit has been weakened and threatened by the changes of the modern technological age. We also have very sophisticated means of communication. Apart from the over-exposure of news through the television networks and the newspapers, we now have personal fax machines, e.mail and the internet, not to mention mobile phones. This means that we can be reached no matter where we are, and because of the power of instant communication, we are obliged to give instant answers. All of this produces more stress in people's lives because of pressure and demand.

Causes of Stress

Stress at work

Many of the stresses at work are caused by overload, underload, role ambiguity, the threat of redundancy and lack of job satisfaction. The fact that there are no longer 'jobs for life' and most contracts are now short-term, has created a huge amount of insecurity, and many families experience instability in their income. Mortgages, however, continue to rise and create, in their wake, a tidal wave of stress and anxiety. Many companies employ stress managers, or stress counsellors to help combat the increasing amount of absenteeism caused by stress and strain. It is thought that sickness through stress costs industry millions of pounds each year and is increasing.

To help soothe work worries, keep an aromatherapy essence burner on your desk, and try a blend of four drops of frankincense and four drops of geranium, or four drops of basil and four drops of bergamot. If you can't use a burner, put the oils on a cotton wool pad and inhale frequently; you can also use this formula as a regular bath oil. Regular aromatherapy massage, using marjoram and lavender in a base oil, will help to release muscular tension and impart well-being.

Before choosing oils check cautionary notes if you have a medical condition, epileptic, or pregnant.

Stress at home

Apart from the stress that is transferred from work to home, stress at home is caused by the lack of finances, disputes with neighbours, problems with the family, children, and illness. There is also another serious cause of stress in the home called, 'I've got the builders in'. Having work done inside or outside the house is one of the greatest stresses of all time, with the exception of moving.

To keep calm amongst the noise of radios, skips, rubble and dust, not to mention making the endless cups of tea, try a blend of four drops of camomile, four drops of lavender, or four drops of neroli and four drops of frankincense. Keep your essence burner going all the time you are exposed to the upheaval. Lemongrass is also a calming and uplifting oil to use.

Personality and stress

Certain personality types have a predisposition to stress, in particular, 'Type A' personalities have been recognised by psychologists as being more likely to suffer with stress-related conditions such as high blood pressure and heart attacks than other personality types. 'Type A' personalities are aggressive, try to over-achieve in everything they do, are always working and forcing themselves toward unrealistic goals, needing to be in control and always aiming to be superior to others. Desperate always to be on time, they are clock-watchers who rush everywhere, are quick to become angry and irritated, cynical, impatient of fools and constantly interrupt or finish your sentences. 'Type A' take on and try to accomplish too much, they walk, talk and eat too quickly.

'Type B' personalities are relaxed, unhurried, non-aggressive, calm and uncompetitive. To become a 'Type B' personality, try a blend of four drops of sandalwood and four drops of ylang ylang, or four drops of vetiver and four drops of bergamot, in a burner, bath or massage oil. Use this blend on a regular basis to avoid some of the symptoms of 'Type A' folk.

Pain and stress

Being in pain from an injury, condition or illness is another cause of stress, and one that cannot be dealt with by changing your attitudes or behaviour. The experience of constant pain is debilitating and causes impatience and irritability. Depending on the condition or illness, aromatherapy massage can help with pain control, but professional help is advisable.

A blend of lavender, camomile and marjoram will help relieve stress and pain. Try three drops in a bath, or five drops of each in 30 ml of base oil. Try the same blend in a burner to bring overall calm and well-being.

Social causes

Some of the other causes of everyday stress are environmental and social. Issues affecting where we live and how we live are, in many cases, out of our control, for example the building of supermarkets in residential areas, the altering of traffic flow, political changes, even the changes brought about by the Europe Union – these are all strong issues which may cause anger, frustration and conflict. The lack of law and order constantly threatens communities, especially some housing estates where youths are allowed to run riot.

For general relaxation, bergamot, lavender and ylang ylang are effective in calming a troubled mind.

Stress and children

Children are not exempt from stress and anxiety, especially at school. They can experience bullying, pressure from exams, peer pressure and competitiveness. Children are also prone to anxiety-related symptoms when exposed to stress via their parents and other family members. A stressed home environment will predispose a child to become a stressed adult.

Try a blend of two drops of Roman camomile and two drops of bergamot to ease anger and irritability. For pre-exam nerves and to aid concentration, try a blend of three drops of basil and three drops of sweet orange or lemongrass in a burner in the study room or generally around the house. The aroma of this blend will help everyone relax and stay calm.

Some of the causes of negative stress responses are usually the small unimportant things that can be described as simply 'the straws that broke the camel's back', and these invariably occur when you have been coping with stress for too long and something just triggers off an outburst. Anyone who happens to be in the way will come under fire, even the cat.

To avoid outbursts that will affect the rest of the family, it is helpful to release tension either by physical exercise such as walking, cycling, swimming, gardening, or a work-out at the gym. The Japanese are encouraged to use punch bags at work to release tension. If you don't possess the real thing, try punching a couple of pillows or cushions instead, but make sure the cat is not curled up and peacefully asleep on them.

208

Then try a blend of four drops of clary sage and four drops of jasmine either in a burner or relaxing bath to bring about the calm after the storm.

Effects of stress

Short-term effects of stress are edginess, insomnia, niggling headaches, itchy skin, muscle tension and irritability.

Long-term stress is more harmful and has been linked with diabetes, heart conditions, high blood pressure, palpitations, high cholesterol levels, eczema, psoriasis, irritable bowel syndrome, bladder problems, asthma, headaches and migraine. Whilst many of these conditions are attributed to genetic and environmental causes, many are triggered solely by stress and anxiety.

Recognising and Managing Stress

Recognising the signs of harmful stress is usually easy when observing the behaviour of someone else; it is more difficult, however, to recognise your own. Some of the signs are uncontrolled irritability and anger, chronic fatigue, regular and excessive drinking, smoking, over-eating, including eating disorders, panic attacks, obsessive behaviour, depression and insomnia: any condition, in fact, that makes a person feel agitated, uncomfortable and demotivated.

To manage any stress, first you must identify the main cause: is it work or home? It might be both. Try to isolate one particular thing that causes stress and establish why this makes you unhappy. We all take our feelings and transfer them to various parts of our life. We take our stress and anxieties from home to work. We then take our work stress and anxiety to home and transfer it to the family. Eventually the stressors from both environments fuse together, causing breakdowns in communication and relationships and resulting in ill-health and unhappiness.

Aromatherapy is one of the best methods of relaxation and stress management, regularly appearing in the media as a way to better health. Used in conjunction with some of the techniques of stress management found in this chapter, it will change your responses to negative stress. It must be emphasised, however, that if you are suffering from clinical depression (see page 51) or severe stress symptoms and you suspect that your overall mental health is in danger, you should seek medical advice.

Prioritising

Prioritising tasks is a classic method of stress management. Make a list of everything you think you have to do. Then apply the 'Four Ds' treatment: look at each task in turn and see which of these 'D' categories it belongs to.

- Do it – it's important, so don't procrastinate, get it over and done with.
- Delay it – this is something that can be put on hold for a while.
- Delegate it – remember, you don't have to do everything, so if someone else can do it, ask them!
- Dump it – there are some things on everyone's lists that really don't need doing.

Even without prioritising, just writing lists is a classic method of stress management which will help put you in control of your life. Each day, write a list of things you have to do, in order of important (use the Four Ds approach, if necessary). Having made your list, get on with the tasks and don't allow anything to distract you. If distractions are unavoidable (and most aren't), then do a couple of smaller jobs from the bottom of the list so that you will at least have the satisfaction of achieving something.

If you are constantly distracted for one reason or another, take a look at your motivation: is it that you really don't want to do any of the tasks – are you, in fact, allowing yourself to be distracted, or are you motivated by a need to please others? Are you unable to say 'No'? Saying 'No' is also an important stress management technique but many people find it hard to do and so fall into the trap of sublimating their own needs to those of other people.

Assertiveness

Learning to say 'No' requires assertiveness skills; assertiveness is all about understanding and meeting your own rights and needs, whilst still respecting those of other people. It isn't about winning or losing, it's about moving and shifting a situation so that the outcome is beneficial to all parties. Assertiveness is not about being aggressive, it means establishing grounds so that you are not compromised or manipulated by guilt, emotional blackmail or pressure. Used skilfully, assertiveness will reduce stress experienced in the home and workplace. To help strengthen assertiveness and build character and resolve, try a blend of two drops frankincense, two drops of geranium and two drops of sandalwood. Use in a burner, bath or massage oil.

Time management

Time management is also helpful in controlling stress, and short courses and books are available on the subject. A simple time management technique is to keep a daily log of the things you have done, how long they have taken, and whether they were part of your daily list (see Prioritising). This way you will see where you have wasted time, procrastinated or allowed yourself to be distracted.

To help avoid procrastination, try a blend of four drops of grapefruit and four drops of sandalwood or cajeput.

Stress and strain, in some instances, cannot be avoided. The type of jobs people do, for example police work and nursing may be stressful by their very nature, and most stress control techniques are pretty useless in many of the situations that arise. Therefore maintaining a regular programme of relaxation is very important if you are in a difficult job or relationship that you do not wish to leave. Many life situations do not allow for the person to change things, so it is very important to have the resources and knowledge to be able to manage and survive.

To help persevere in difficult circumstances, try a blend of four drops of frankincense and four drops of sandalwood.

Because negative stress is based on how we perceive things to be, life can be improved by changing your perception, which in turn will help you to respond differently. Stress occurs when the demands of a situation seem to be greater than the resources we have available to cope with the problem. We often approach a situation or task from the end result, rather than the starting post. We see it as overwhelming and say to ourselves, even before we start, 'I can't cope with this'. Many years ago, my stress management tutor asked me how I would eat an elephant. I replied, 'One bite at a time, unless of course it was a chocolate one!' 'That is how you approach an overwhelming task or situation', she said, 'One step at a time'. I have used this approach many times since then and it works very well.

You can also try using the 'ants and elephants' technique: each day take one or two bites at your elephant (large tasks) and eat as many ants (smaller tasks) as you can. This helps achieve goals without added pressure.

To help your appetite for ants and elephants, try burning a blend of four drops of basil and four drops of lavender.

Depression

Depression is a serious symptom of stress; it is that feeling when everything seems pointless and hopeless; a state of confusion, gloom and an overwhelming feeling of inadequacy. Depression is usually triggered by situations and events beyond our control and gradually destroys our spirit and vitality. It takes time and understanding to deal with depression and the related illness, clinical depression. Clinical depression is caused by an imbalance of neuro chemicals in the brain, affecting our moods, and behaviour. It is a serious condition and sufferers require medical help. Depression can also be hormone-related, as in the menopause, and can cause problems during this time of life. Depression caused by stress or the menopause can be greatly helped by using aromatherapy and other alternative therapies, but also by simply talking to a trusted friend. It is not a time to allow self-pity to control your emotions, neither is it a time to beat yourself up because you are feeling depressed: it is a time to take action and try each day to take one step forward. As you achieve progress, praise yourself to the hilt for being brave and courageous, and at the end of each week give yourself a present. Pamper yourself with an aromatherapy treatment to keep boosting your flagging spirits.

Try a blend of four drops of jasmine and four drops of bergamot. See also suggested oils on page 167. Marjoram is not suitable for clinical depression.

Fatigue

Fatigue is another insidious sympton of stress; in fact it is the first sign of the just-coping syndrome, when instead of feeling in control of our lives, we see barely coping as the norm. It overwhelms both mind and body and the feeling is one of being disconnected from any energy at all. Fatigue is entirely different from the tiredness you feel after a hard day's work, or even a hard day's fun. When you have worked hard or played hard, you are restored by a good night's sleep, whereas stress fatigue never goes away. You wake up feeling tired, and this tired feeling continues until you go to bed at night.

Massage is an excellent remedy for both depression and fatigue, as it stimulates the production of endorphins. These are chemicals produced by the brain that bind to our pain receptors, similar in action to the drug morphine. The production of endorphins helps to relax muscles and create a feeling of well-being. Gentle, pleasant exercise will also aid recovery from depression and the lifting of fatigue.

To dispel physical and mental fatigue, try a blend of four drops of rosemary (see cautions on page 102) and four drops of frankincense. Substitute grapefruit if you have high blood pressure.

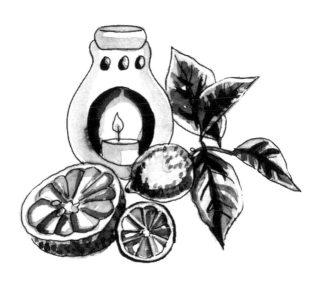

Oils to Relieve Stress

Some of the essential oils that are particularly helpful to stress conditions are:

BASIL
Strengthens the nervous system and relieves mental fatigue.

BERGAMOT
Relaxes and releases the body and mind from the strains of the day, leaving a floaty feeling of well-being; it is also an anti-depressant.

CAMOMILE (ROMAN)
Helps with feelings of frustration and anger; it is soothing to both mind and body and is also an anti-depressant.

CLARY SAGE
Helps with panic attacks, depression and relaxation, and restores energy.

FRANKINCENSE
Lifts fatigue and restores energy, imparts a feeling of strength and well-being.

JASMINE
Helps lift depression and is very calming and soothing.

LAVENDER
Helps in all areas of stress, anxiety and worry.

MARJORAM
Helps with feelings of hopelessness and loneliness, which can be caused by stress; also lifts depression. (Please note, however, that marjoram should be avoided if you are being treated with medication for depression, as it can have a stupefying effect, and would be contra-indicated with the use of tranquillisers.)

NEROLI
Calming, relaxing and uplifting.

ROSE
Heals the heart energy, and will be effective in treating all types of stress-related conditions.

SANDALWOOD
Effective in soothing the mind from troubled thoughts, uplifting to depression.

VETIVER
Makes an effective, deeply relaxing massage oil, beneficial for all effects of stress.

YLANG YLANG
Calms and soothes both mind and body, helping to calm palpitations caused by stress.

This is not the definitive list of oils to help with your stress management programme, so do look under each individual listing in Chapter 7. However, the oils I have highlighted here are particularly good and will complement each other when several are blended together.

For most effective results, use essential oils regularly several times a week, by either massage, bathing or in an essence burner. The expenditure on the oils and equipment will be repaid many times over as you feel the changes occurring in your mind, body and spirit.

Suggested Reading

AROMATHERAPY

Patricia Davis, *Aromatherapy: an A–Z*, CW Daniel & Co., 1988.

Marcel Lavabre, *Aromatherapy Workbook*, Healing Arts Press, Vermont, 1990.

Julia Lawless, *The Encyclopaedia of Essential Oils*, Element Books, 1992.

Gabriel Mojay, *Aromatherapy Healing the Spirit*, Gaia Books Ltd, 1996.

Danielle Ryman, *The Encyclopaedia of Plant Oils and How They Help You*, Piatkus Books, 1991.

Wanda Sellar, *The Directory of Essential Oils*, CW Daniel & Co., 1992.

Valerie Ann Worwood, *The Fragrant Pharmacy*, Macmillan, 1990.

Valerie Ann Worwood, *The Fragrant Mind*, Doubleday, 1995.

MASSAGE

Nigel Dawes and Fiona Harrold, *Massage Cures*, Thorsons, 1990.

Clare Maxwell-Hudson, *The Complete Book of Massage*, Dorling Kindersley.

REFLEXOLOGY

Ann Gillanders, *Reflexology: The Ancient Answer to Modern Ailments*, Jenny Lee Publishing, 1987.

SELF GROWTH

Louise L Hay, *The Power is Within You*, Eden Grove Editions, 1991.

Louise L Hay, *You Can Heal Your Life*, Eden Grove Editions, 1984.

Florence Scovell Shinn, *The Game of Life and How to Play It,* 39th edition, LN Fowler & Co., 1991.

Bernie Siegal MD, *Love, Medicine and Miracles,* Arrow Books, 1986.

Bernie Siegal MD, *Peace, Love and Healing,* Rider, 1990.

Andrew Mathews, *Being Happy,* Media Masters, 1995.

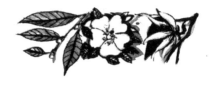

Reputable Suppliers

Mail order specialists for true essential oils, base oils, creams and lotions, massage oils and aromatherapy products.

DeFraine Aromatic Oils
Lavender House
13 Carlton Road
Sidcup
Kent DA14 6AQ
Tel/Fax 0181 302 1946

Butterbur and Sage Ltd
7 Tessa Road
Reading
Berks RG1 8HH
Tel 0118 950 5100

Aromatherapy Associates
68 Maltings Place
Bagleys Lane
London SW6 2BY
Tel 0171 371 9878, Fax 0171 371 9894

Shirley Price Aromatherapy
Essentia House
Upper Bond Street
Hinckley
Leicestershire LE10 1RS
Tel 0455 615466, Fax 0455 615054

Associations

AOC (Aromatherapy Organisations Council)
3 Latymer Close
Braybrooke
Market Harborough
Leicestershire LE16 8LN
Tel/Fax 01858 434242

IFA (International Federation of Aromatherapists)
Stamford House
2–4 Chiswick High Road
London W4 1TH
Tel 0181 742 2605

ISPA (International Society of Professional Aromatherapists)
ISPA House
82 Ashby Road
Hinchley
Leicestershire LE10 1SN
Tel 01455 637987

IFA and ISPA will supply details of training courses and qualified practitioners. For a full list of associations and courses write to AOC (address above).

Joan Radford is available to hold lectures, seminars, workshops and courses in aromatherapy, stress management, self-development, spiritual awareness and emotional healing.
Tel/Fax 0181 302 1946

About the Author

JOAN Radford discovered the benefits of aromatherapy in 1979 after having had both physical and emotional problems due to overweight and eating disorders. With regular aromatherapy massage, her stress-related symptoms were soon under control and she began to see her life in a more balanced way. This, in turn, helped her cope with and cure the eating disorder. Because aromatherapy had been so effective in her recovery, Joan decided to take it up professionally, and successfully qualified in Massage, Aromatherapy and Relexology in 1981. Since that time, she has worked continuously in her very successful private practice. She has become one of the most skilled, sought-after and busiest aromatherapists in the profession.

Joan has worked extensively with people with learning difficulties and special needs at a day centre in Bromley Kent, and in 1987 set up a training programme for the staff which has now been taken up by other day-care centres.

A qualified teacher and an accomplished lecturer, Joan has conducted courses in the UK, Israel and the United States on aromatherapy, stress, stress-related symptoms and the emotional links to disease. The success of the courses prompted Joan to take up stress management and personal development as another branch of her work. She is now a qualified stress manager and holds a distinction in this field.

During her career, Joan has been chairperson of the Holistic Aromatherapy Foundation, executive officer for the Aromatherapy Organisations Council, and a consultant for several essential oil companies. She has been featured in magazine and newspaper articles as well as radio interviews.

Index

disinfectants 70
distillation 12, 14, 16, 25–6
diverticulitis 75
dyspepsia *see* indigestion

earache 63
effleurage 113
elderly 49, 63, 65, 106, 147–51, 180
emotions/mood 76, 78, 91, 162, 195–202
emphysema 73
enfleurage 15
epileptics 49, 83, 84
essence burners 65–8
essential oils
    accidents with 52–3
    adulteration 18, 41–3
    adverse reactions 46, 48, 52–3, 54, 108
    availability/price 38
    base/middle/top notes 34, 35–6
    blending 26, 27, 36
    frequency of use 53–4, 58
    internal/external use 8
    labelling 43–4
    methods of use 57–71
    neat 69
    organic 39–40
    phototoxicity 54, 86, 91, 92
    properties 20–3, 72–109
    purity 40
    storing 37, 44, 57
    synergistic 26
    toxicity 53, 54–6
eucalyptus 26, 83
European Union 39, 43
exhaustion *see fatigue*
expression method 16

face oils 58–6
fainting 170
fatigue 60, 61, 128, 151, 169, 213–14
    mental 61, 86, 150

fear 84, 85, 99, 101, 197–8, 200, 203
fennel 3–4, 31
fibrositis 170
first aid 170
flatulence 21, 84
fleas 70
fluid retention (oedema) 97, 102, 133, 171
foot conditions 82, 171–2
frankincense 38, 84–5, 134–5, 138–9
fungal nail infections 69

garlic 71
Gattefosse, R-M. 12–13
geranium 35, 85, 131–4
ginger 86
glandular fever 172
gout 73, 88, 102, 173
grapefruit 86–7, 131–4
grapeseed oil 47, 59, 153
grief/anguish 150, 173
guilt 174, 201
gum disease 91, 95, 107

haemorrhoids 62, 174
hair conditioners 62
halitosis *see* mouthwashes
handicapped people 50
hangovers 63
hazelnut oil 47
headaches/migraines 145, 175–6, 183–4
    compresses 63, 64
    essential oils 69, 90, 91, 93, 102
    massage 116
    reflexology 126
herbal medicine 25–6
holistic approach 13, 27, 195–202
hormone replacement therapy (HRT) 50, 81, 182
hormones 31, 84, 85, 101, 137
hyssop 22

immune system 23, 50, 106, 172